Ultrasound and Infertility

Editor

Asim Kurjak, M.D., Ph.D.

Professor and Chairman
Ultrasonic Institute
Collaborative Center for Diagnostic Ultrasound
World Health Organization
Zagreb, Yugoslavia

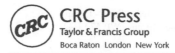
CRC Press
Taylor & Francis Group
Boca Raton London New York

CRC Press is an imprint of the
Taylor & Francis Group, an **informa** business

CRC Press
Taylor & Francis Group
6000 Broken Sound Parkway NW, Suite 300
Boca Raton, FL 33487-2742

© 1989 by Taylor & Francis Group, LLC
CRC Press is an imprint of Taylor & Francis Group, an Informa business

First issued in paperback 2019

No claim to original U.S. Government works

ISBN 13: 978-0-367-45108-0 (pbk)
ISBN 13: 978-0-8493-4766-5 (hbk)

**Visit the Taylor & Francis Web site at
http://www.taylorandfrancis.com**

**and the CRC Press Web site at
http://www.crcpress.com**

Library of Congress Card Number 88-14469

Library of Congress Cataloging-in-Publication Data

Ultrasound and infertility /editor, Asim Kurjak.
     p.   cm.
   Includes bibliographies and index.
   ISBN 0-8493-4766-1
   1. Infertility — Diagnosis. 2. Generative organs — Ultrasonic imaging.   I. Kurjak, Asim.
   [DNLM: 1. Infertility — diagnosis. 2. Infertility — therapy. 3. Ultrasonic Diagnosis. 4. Ultrasonic Therapy. WP 570 U47]
RC889.U37 1989
618.1′7207543 — dc19
DNLM/DLC
for Library of Congress   88-14469
                                                                                        CIP

PREFACE

It has been more than 30 years since the late Professor Ian Donald first started to use ultrasound in obstetrics and gynecology. In a relatively short period of time, ultrasound has improved in what seems to be a logarithmic progression, and it can, with good reason, be said to have changed the way of thinking of modern obstetricians.

However, until recently, the progress was not so rapid in the field of infertility; but, in the last 10 years, ultrasound has become a highly sophisticated scientific tool readily available for the diagnosis and management of infertile couples. Ultrasound has a permanent advantage over other imaging and diagnostic techniques by being rapid, safe, and noninvasive. Therefore, ultrasound is being used with increasing success to determine the time of ovulation, artificial insemination, or *in vitro* fertilization.

In addition, ultrasound appears to be a safe, practical, and noninvasive alternative to laparoscopy in many aspects. It is, therefore, time to produce a book which will serve as a useful guide for the optimal use of ultrasound in an infertility clinic, containing most of the information necessary for practical work, and bringing ultrasonographers and clinicians up to date information on the current knowledge and special problems for the future.

Asim Kurjak

THE EDITOR

Asim Kurjak, M.D., Ph.D., is chairman of the department and professor of Obstetrics and Gynecology at the University of Zagreb, Yugoslavia. He is also head of the Ultrasonic Institute of Zagreb which is the World Health Organization Collaborative Center for diagnostic ultrasound.

Dr. Kurjak obtained his training at the University of Zagreb, receiving his M.D. degree in 1966 and his Ph.D. degree in 1977. He served as an assistant professor at the Department of Obstetrics and Gynecology, University of Zagreb from 1968 to 1980. In 1971, as a British scholar, he was research assistant for 1 year at the Institute of Obstetrics and Gynecology, University of London. From 1983 to 1985 he was external examiner at the University of Liverpool. It was in 1983 that he assumed his present position.

Dr. Kurjak is a member and past president of the Yugoslav Society of University Professors Academy of Croatia. He is member of the advisory board of four international scientific journals. He served as vice president of the European federation for ultrasound in medicine and biology. He has been the recipient of many research grants from the Scientific Council from Yugoslavia and is currently the WHO coordinator for the use of ultrasound in developing countries. Among other awards, he is an honorary member of Ultrasonic Society of Australia, Italia, Egypt, Indonesia and of the Sociation of Obstetrics and Gynecology of Italia, Poland, and Hungary.

Dr. Kurjak has presented over 70 invited lectures at major international meetings and approximately 100 guest lectures at universities and institutes. He has published more than 200 research papers and 14 books in the English language. His current major research interests include ultrasound diagnosis and fetal and Doppler studies of fetoplacental and maternal blood flow.

CONTRIBUTORS

Marinko Biljan, M.D.
Ultrasonic Institute
Medical Faculty
University of Zagreb
Zagreb, Yugoslavia

Menashe Ben-David, Ph.D.
Department of Obstetrics & Gynecology
Hadassah University Hospital
Jerusalem, Israel

Branko Breyer, Ph.D.
Head
Medical Physics Department
Gynecological Cancer Center
University Gynecological Hospital
Zagreb, Yugoslavia

Zeljko Fuchkar, M.D., Ph.D.
Associate Professor
Urology and Kidney Transplants
Clinical Hospital Center
Faculty of Medicine
University "Vladimir Bakaric"
Rijeka, Yugoslavia

Davor Jurkovic, M.D.
Research Fellow
Ultrasonic Institute
Medical Faculty
University of Zagreb
Zagreb, Yugoslavia

Asim Kurjak, M.D., Ph.D.
Professor and Chairman
Ultrasonic Institute
Collaborative Center for Diagnostic
 Ultrasound
World Health Organization
Zagreb, Yugoslavia

Aby Lewin, M.D.
Department of Obstetrics & Gynecology
Hadassah University Hospital
Jerusalem, Israel

Shraga Rottem, M.D.
Department of Obstetrics & Gynecology
Rambam Medical Center
Medical School
Technion-Institute of Technology
Haifa, Israel

Joseph G. Schenker, M.D.
Professor and Chairman
Department of Obstetrics & Gynecology
Hadassah University Hospital
Jerusalem, Israel

Ilan E. Timor-Tritsch, M.D.
Professor and Director
Department of Obstetrics & Gynecology
College of Physicians & Surgeons
Columbia University
New York, New York

TABLE OF CONTENTS

Chapter 1

BASIC PHYSICS OF ULTRASOUND

Branko Breyer

TABLE OF CONTENTS

I. INTRODUCTION

In this chapter, we describe the basic physical and technological principles of ultrasound diagnostics without mathematical treatment, except for some simple formulas, yet include comments relevant for practical use. Ultrasound diagnostic instruments and procedures are still in fast development, so that mere knowledge of manipulation with the existing instruments is definitely insufficient for sound usage of the existing instruments to come in a few years. The knowledge of underlying principles allows one to understand what is actually new in an instrument, and what are the supposed advantages.

II. PHYSICAL PRINCIPLES

A. Ultrasound Waves

Ultrasound is, per definition, the sound of a frequency higher than the hearing limit of the human ear, i.e., above 16 to 20 kHz. Bat's definition of ultrasound would be different. In medical diagnostics, one normally uses ultrasound waves of frequencies between 2 and 10 MHz. Basic physical principles are equally valid for audible sound as for ultrasound, only at different scales. Ultrasound is a mechanical wave, i.e., it consists of mechanical vibrations of medium particles through which it propagates. In soft tissues, the medium particles vibrate along the direction of wave propagation creating their densifications and rarefactions in space. Such a wave is called a longitudinal wave. The particles (molecules) oscillate around their (stochastic) balance positions with no net flow of matter, however, the energy flows. At very high energy densities some net flow can be induced, but this does not apply to energies of ultrasound used in diagnostics. Other types of waves like transversal and Raileigh cannot propagate to any appreciable distance in soft tissues. Ultrasound waves are characterized by parameters like frequency, wavelength, propagation speed, intensity, and pressure. Frequency is expressed in hertz (Hz), i.e., cycles per second. The physical dimension is 1/s; 1 Hz = 1 c/s, 1 kHz = 1000 c/s, and 1 MHz = 1 million c/s. The frequency used in diagnostics largely influences their properties. Wavelength is the distance between the same phases of compression of the medium in two consecutive cycles in space and is measured in meters or its subunits like millimeters. The propagation speed depends mainly on the media (tissue) properties through which the wave propagates and is related with frequency and wavelength as follows:

$$\lambda = \frac{c}{f}$$

where c = propagation velocity in meters per second (m/s), f = frequency in hertz (Hz), and λ = wavelength in meters (m).

Strictly speaking, sounds of different frequencies travel at different velocities (frequency velocity dispersion), but these effects are negligible at frequencies, intensities, and circumstances of medical echography. The average propagation speed in soft tissues is 1540 m/s. The speed depends on both density and elastic properties of tissues.

When traveling through tissues, ultrasound causes a variation of the total pressure, i.e., the sonic pressure oscillations are superimposed upon the static pressure (atmospheric pressure). The measure of energy density flowing through a unity area in one unit of time is called intensity and is expressed in watts per square meter or centimeter (W/cm^2 or W/m^2).

When speaking about ultrasound intensity in an ultrasound beam, it is not sufficient to simply state the intensity, one must as well state "where" and "when"; i.e., at what position in space and within which interval. Simply stating the intensity applies only to a plane wave in a nonattenuating medium. In echography, one uses pulsed ultrasound and focused beams

Table 1
ORIENTATIONAL VALUES
OF PROPAGATION SPEEDS
IN SOFT TISSUES[1,2]

Tissue	Speed (m/s)
Muscle	1570
Kidney	1560
Liver	1560
Brain	1510
Fat	1440

Note: The speed values are for orientation only. Inspection of the available literature shows fairly divergent results. There is a consensus that the average speed for soft tissues should be taken as 1540 m/s.

in attenuating media. After we discuss characteristics of ultrasound beams, we shall turn back to definitions of ultrasound intensities in the beam.

Likewise, when speaking about frequency, one can define a single frequency only as a continuous wave. When speaking about pulses of some frequency, we usually think of frequency obtained by counting the number of zero-level crossings during the pulse. However, a pulse by physical laws contains a mixture of frequencies which we call the frequency spectrum of the pulse, and which is broader — the shorter the pulse. This fact must be born in mind in the practical use of ultrasound echography because, as we shall show, one uses different frequencies for different purposes, so it may sometimes be useful to bear in mind that when using, e.g., a probe declared 3.5 MHz central frequency, one actually transmits and receives a spectrum of frequencies, which may range from below 1 MHz to more than 5 MHz.

B. Ultrasound Propagation in Tissues

Human tissues are not homogenous in respect to ultrasound wave propagation, so that in transversing the tissues, ultrasound waves are being reflected, refracted, scattered, and absorbed. Angle of refraction depends on the respective velocities in the tissues.

The amount of reflected energy depends on characteristic acoustic impedances and angle of incidence upon the boundary of tissues. The tissues we are speaking about are different tissues in terms of elasticity and other physical properties, but can be parts of the same biological tissue. Characteristic acoustic impedance is a property of a medium and is defined as the ratio of the momentary acoustic pressure and particle velocity induced by this pressure.

In different tissues, ultrasound velocities and impedance are generally different (see Table 1). Differences between different soft tissues are much smaller than between soft tissues and bones, respectively, gas. This fact has important consequences in the use of ultrasound in medicine.

1. Refraction and Reflection of Ultrasound Waves

In discussing reflection and refraction of ultrasound, we shall take the simplest case — the plane wave — which, although an idealization, will give us a good idea of what happens when ultrasound waves transverse a boundary of media which is much larger than the wavelength.

As illustrated in Figure 1, a part of the energy is reflected and some of the energy is

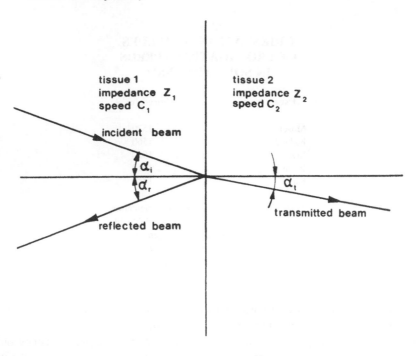

FIGURE 1.   Reflection and refraction of ultrasound waves on a media boundary. The two media have different characteristic impedances (Z_1 and Z_2) and different propagation speeds (c_1 and c_2). The boundary dimensions are larger than the wavelength.

transmitted across the boundary. The angle of refraction depends on the ratio of propagation speeds in the two respective media, as described by Equation 1, while the refraction of energy reflected depends on the difference of characteristic acoustic impedances, as well as on the angle of incidence. (Equation 2a). If the speeds of ultrasound in the first and the second medium are c_1 and c_2, respectively, and the incidence angle is α_i and the transmission angle is α_t, then the refraction angle can be calculated from Equation 1:

$$\frac{\sin\alpha_i}{\sin\alpha_t} = \frac{c_1}{c_2} \tag{1}$$

Equation 2 describes the ratio of the amplitudes of the reflected and the incident wave:

$$\frac{A_r}{A_i} = \frac{Z_2 \cos\alpha_i - Z_1 \cos\alpha_t}{Z_2 \cos\alpha_i + Z_1 \cos\alpha_t} \tag{2a}$$

If the incidence is perpendicular to the media boundary, Equation 2a degenerates to

$$\frac{A_r}{A_i} = \frac{Z_2 - Z_1}{Z_2 + Z_1} \tag{2b}$$

In many practical cases when we consider ultrasound waves, which are reflected back to the transmitting probe, Equation 2b gives a fairly accurate picture of what goes on.

Intensity of ultrasound is proportional to the square of its pressure so that the ratio of the reflected to the incident intensity is at 90°

$$\frac{I_r}{I_i} = \frac{(Z_2 - Z_1)^2}{(Z_2 + Z_1)^2} \tag{3}$$

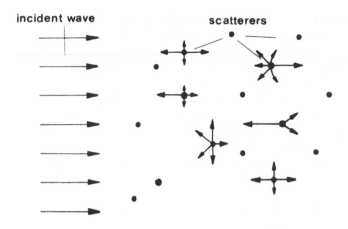

FIGURE 2. The incident waves encounter scatterers stochastically dispersed in the medium. The incident waves induce oscillations of the scatterers, which retransmit wavelets in varied directions with different intensities (illustrated by arrow lengths). The waves that are backscattered add up and interfere, and as such, are detected by the receiving transducer.

If the characteristic acoustic impedances are very different like in the case of soft tissue and gas (e.g., in lungs), from the above equation one can see that virtually all ultrasound energy will be reflected. A consequence of this is that organs containing gas, such as the lungs, cannot be examined by ultrasound, and gas in the stomach and intestines will present serious problems. Another consequence is that some sort of contact gel, oil, or other coupling agent should be applied between the ultrasound transmitter and the body to avoid air bubbles being trapped between the probe and the skin and to allow ultrasound to enter the body. It is interesting to see that ultrasound will be reflected irrespective of whether it enters from a lower or a higher impedance. The absolute value of reflected wave is the same for the same difference in characteristic acoustic impedances. On the other hand, the sign changes indicate a difference in phase.

The energy that is not reflected will be transmitted across the impedance boundary. Thus, in many cases it is the characteristic acoustic impedance that is decisive for the intensity of an echo. Sometimes the acoustic impedance is mixed up with the density by a vague analogy with X-ray imaging. This is wrong because the characteristic impedance depends on the density and propagation speed (c):

$$Z = \rho \cdot c$$

and not only on the density.

So far we have considered the situation illustrated in Figure 1 where the impedance boundary is continuous and much larger than the wavelength. Such a reflector is called specular, i.e., mirror-like. There are many structures in the body which act as specular reflectors, but there are even more structures in which the reflectors are of dimensions similar or smaller than the wavelength. Such small reflectors scatter ultrasound in different directions similar to what happens when light is shined through a sheet of paper. Figure 2 illustrates what happens with ultrasound waves when transversing tissues such as the liver and muscles and many other tissues in the body.

The wavelets from scatterers are retransmitted in all directions and add up in different, only stochastically predictable ways. They interfere among themselves, and the resulting waves that return to the transmitting probe do not exactly represent each of the scatterers. This has important consequences on our interpretation of echographic images (Table 1).

As one can see from Table 1 the speed of ultrasound in different tissues varies, which introduces certain errors in distance measurements. In the majority of cases, this is not very important and one usually settles for an average calibration speed of 1540 m/s for soft tissues. In some instances, this is not good enough and then the problem is circumvented by agreeing upon a standard calibration velocity (e.g., 1540 or 1600 m/s), then measuring the normal dimension of interest using this calibration velocity, and finally producing a graph or table containing normal values with the above supposition. Later on, one can compare values obtained by measurement with the normals, and not with the inaccesible, real values. In this way, one can tell whether or not a dimension is normal (bone length, biparietal diameter, etc.), which is what we really need, but one can be by some percentage wrong when comparing the actual, inaccessible dimension, which is not really important.

Absorption of ultrasound in tissues reduces ultrasound intensity as it passes through the tissues. Attenuation is further increased by the scattering of ultrasound waves. Both phenomena are frequency dependent and are expressed more at higher frequencies. Therefore, higher frequency ultrasound beams are more readily attenuated than the lower frequency beams and so, when we need to scan deeper structures, we must apply lower frequency ultrasound. At present, one typically uses approximately 3 MHz for general abdominal scanning in adults (liver, pancreas, advanced pregnancy); and about 5 MHz for children scanning, early pregnancy, neck, and breast; and 7 MHz for shallow scanning. A general rule is that the highest frequency will still satisfy penetration; i.e., the shortest applicable wavelength should be used.

Apart from this, scattering, absorption, and velocity are characteristic of tissues and are potential means of quantitatively characterizing tissues. Many experiments are under way along these lines with a fair probability that they will lead to quantitative ways of describing and diagnosing diffuse lesions of parenchymatous organs and differentiating malignant from benign lesions or at least stating a heavy suspicion of malignancy.

III. ECHOSCOPIC SYSTEMS

Ultrasound waves can be used, for medical diagnostics, in many different ways, but the most common method at present is ultrasonic echography. The principle is very simple. One sends out into the body pulses of ultrasound (about 1 μs long) and the echoes from different reflectors and scatterers in the body are detected by the same probe, which was used for transmission. Knowing the speed of ultrasound and measuring the time necessary for the echoes to return, the distance to the reflectors could be calculated. The direction in which the ultrasound pulses have been transmitted is known too, so that one can determine the position of a reflector in two dimensions. The echoes are usually shown on a screen in B, A, or M mode. A and B modes are shown in Figure 3. In A mode (amplitude mode), the echoes returning from along the line of sight of the transmitting receiving probe are shown as peaks proportional to the intensity of reflected ultrasound pulses at their respective depths. While this method of display is nowadays rarely applied, we shall describe it in more detail, because this helps to understand the more complicated and more often used B-mode display. The procedure is as follows: approximately 1000 times per second short pulses are transmitted into the body. Synchronously with the ultrasound pulse transmission, a line begins to be drawn on a cathode-ray tube (CRT) screen. Since the transmitted pulse is only 1 μs long, we have in principle 999 μs at our disposal for registration of echoes. Whenever an echo returns, it is received by the same probe, amplified, and then taken to the CRT tube where the line is deflected proportionally to the returned echo intensity, so that the peak is shown on the screen. The distance between peaks in the screen corresponds to some degree to the actual distance between the reflectors in the body. If the writing velocity at the screen is made exactly half of the speed of ultrasound in the body, the scale will be 1:1,

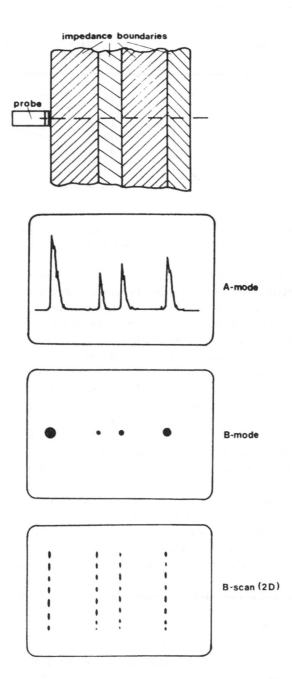

FIGURE 3. An illustration of A- and B-mode displays. Ultrasound pulses reflect from the tissue boundaries and are displayed as peaks or bright dots on the echoscope screen. If the transducer scans the body interior, the resulting bright dots in the B-mode form into a tomographic image of the scanned area.

because ultrasound makes a round trip in the body. This basic method of obtaining an A-mode display in many instances at present has been substituted by more indirect methods, although the principle is the same. The A mode is still used in neurology, ophthalmology, and indirectly in tissue characterization.

In the B-mode display (brightness modulation), the returned echoes are shown as bright

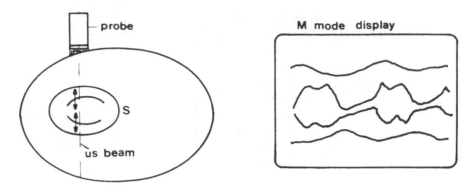

FIGURE 4.   In M-mode display, the still structures are shown as straight lines and the moving ones as wavy lines. The ordinate is the depth and the abscissa is the running time.

dots on the screen. The position of bright dots on the screen corresponds to the position of corresponding reflectors due to the electronic system that measures the time necessary for echoes to return (the round trip time) and the position and angulation of the transmitting-receiving transducer. In real-time systems, which comprise a vast majority of all scanners, the transmitting-receiving probe is automatically moved or angulated, scanning in this way the interior of the body. There are some systems that electronically mimic this movement with the same result of scanning the body. In real-time systems, this ultrasound beam steering is done fast enough to produce a live image. The bright dots (Figure 3) are arrayed in the processor memory and then processed (smoothed, interpolated, etc.) and displayed. The image is a tomographic (section) image of the interior of the body in front of the ultrasound scanning probe. It consists basically of data along the lines corresponding to probe lines of sight. In practice, the section thickness depends on the probe, which we describe in detail later on, and scanner setting too. The thickness in practice range is approximately between 2 and 10 mm.

M mode (movement) is another way of representing ultrasonic echoes, in particular the moving structures. Figure 4 illustrates obtaining an M-mode display. Here too, the echoes are represented by bright dots on the screen, but this time the display is not linked to the system or continuous measurement and determination of transmitting transducer angle, but the transducer is continuously aimed in the same, fixed direction of the moving structure of interest (e.g., heart). The system measures the depths of the moving structures and displays these (changing) depths as they change in time. One axis, usually the abscissa, thus is the running time; the other, usually the ordinate, is the reflector depth. In this way, it is possible to show quantitatively the movement characteristics of, e.g., heart valves, and measure their opening and closing velocities. M-mode display plays an important role in echocardiography, and elaborate methods of detailed processing of data obtained in this way have been developed.

A. Main Blocks of an Echoscope

An echoscope uses short ultrasound pulses to obtain two-dimensional (2D) B-mode images in roughly the following way: short pulses are transmitted from a transmitter-receiver probe into the body. The echoes returning from reflective structures within the body are picked up with the same probe and then electronically processed to obtain a section image on a television (TV) screen. This can be accomplished because, in measuring the time necessary for echoes to return, one knows the velocity of ultrasound along the line of sight or the probe. Echoes that traveled a longer way, return later and are more attenuated. Therefore, the later-coming echoes (echoes coming from deeper structures) must be more amplified in

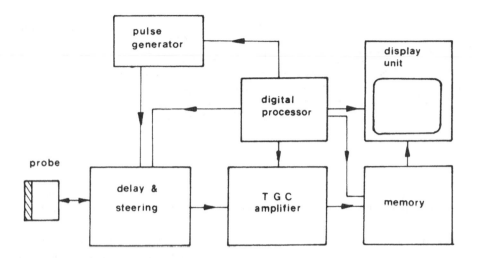

FIGURE 5. Block diagram of an echoscope. A digital processor directs the pulses from a pulse generator via a delay and steering unit into the probe. Signals from the probe (echoes) are processed in the delay unit, taken to the TGC system, amplified, memorized, and prepared for display. The whole process is synchronized and coordinated by the digital processor (computer) and its software.

the echoscope in order to compensate for this attenuation. Such amplified, compensated signals are taken to the digitizing system, which converts the data into a form suitable for digital storage. The procedure is controlled by at least one microprocessor. The content of the microcomputer memory is then displayed on a TV monitor. A simplified block diagram of a system capable of doing this is shown in Figure 5.

The probe is the crucial element of an echoscope and its properties dictate many of the system's characteristics. The probe contains one or more ultrasound transducers. A transducer is a device capable of converting one kind of energy or signal into another kind; in our case, the transducers convert electrical pulses into ultrasonic (mechanical) pulses and vice versa. The same transducers act as transmitters and receivers of ultrasound at different times.

In the beginning of a transmission cycle, the pulse generator generates a very short electrical pulse (tens to some hundreds of volts). This impulse is taken to the transducers in the probe via a control and delay unit, which takes the pulse from the pulse generator to the appropriate transducers in the probe at the appropriate times. After the transmission of the short ultrasound pulse is completed, the system waits for the echoes from the body to return. As the echoes return back to the probe, the transducers pick them up and generate electrical signals, which are now taken to the complicated amplifier, the time gain compensation (TGC) amplifier, which amplifies the signals. The signals that come later are amplified more in order to compensate for attenuation of ultrasound in the body. The amplified signals, which represent reflectors within the body, are stored in a digital memory together with data on the depth and direction they returned from. The depth is inferred from the time interval between the transmission of the pulse and the reception of an echo (taking the average ultrasound propagation speed of 1540 m/s into account). The direction is known from the probe steering data, which are stored in the microprocessor, which controls the scanning procedure. The data from the memory are taken to the display unit and displayed. For various reasons, one cannot simply display all the data as they come from the body, so they are processed before being shown on the screen. The processing always includes some sort of compression of data because the range of ultrasound intensities of interest which return from the body is much larger than the range that can be shown linearly as different brightnesses on a TV screen. On the other hand, different echo intensities are encoded as

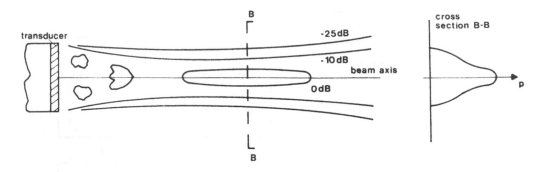

FIGURE 6.   An ultrasonic beam intensity is not uniform or sharply cut off. It can be described with isointensity or isopressure curves. In the focal region it is narrowed. The intensity near the transducer is irregular.

different shades of grey on the screen. This transfer function is therefore nonlinear and can be changed with controls. Apart from this, in modern scanners there regularly is an additional interpolation program, which makes the image better adjusted to human perception characteristics, and in some more sophisticated systems, it mathematically improves the resolution of the details by taking into account some characteristics of the probe and ultrasound propagation through the body.

In the history of ultrasound echography (i.e., only 10 years ago), there was one other type of scanner — the static scanner — which played an important role in obtaining good quality images. These systems, now rare, used a single probe, which was hand moved by the operator with the consequence that the operator had a freedom of choice of the scanning format. The imaging was not real time, but the images were of good quality and with a fixed geometrical relation to the patient couch. The angle and position of the probe were measured by an electromechanical device from which the probe was hanging. At present, these systems are rarely manufactured, so we shall not describe them in detail.

B. Transducer and the Ultrasound Beam

As mentioned above, the transducer converts ultrasound signals into electrical signals and vice versa. The active element of a transducer is a piezoelectric ceramic element or a piezoelectric plastic foil. The property of a piezoelectric material is to deform under the influence of mechanical force (stress), and to generate electrical charge on its sides if it is subjected to mechanical stress. In echography, electrical pulses are taken onto the sides of piezoelectric transducers inducing vibrations in them, which are transmitted into the body as ultrasonic vibrations. Conversely, the echoes from the body induce minute deformations of the transducers so that electrical charge appears at their sides covered with conductive layers from where it is taken to amplifiers in the echoscope.

We must pay more attention to the volume in the medium (water, human body, etc.) which is occupied by this ultrasonic energy and which we call an ultrasonic beam. Figure 6 shows schematically the ultrasonic beam in front of a transducer. It is represented by curves that connect points of equal ultrasound intensity — the isointensity curves. A beam like this can be obtained only in nonattenuating media (degassed water is near enough to this for our purposes). In attenuating media, the actual intensity is modified by attenuation, but the echoscope will "see" an equivalent beam like the one shown in Figure 6 if the TGC amplifier is correctly adjusted.

The intensity is not sharply cut off, but gradually decreases to zero on the sides. If the transducer is focused, then the beam has a narrowing around the focus. Near the transducer, ultrasound intensity is irregular due to interference of ultrasound waves from different parts of the transducer face. Far from the transducer, ultrasound intensity decreases regularly and

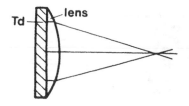

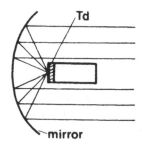

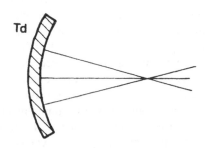

FIGURE 7. Ultrasonic waves can be focused with lenses, mirrors, or curved transducers and combinations thereof.

continuously. The two zones can be mathematically defined. The near zone is called the Fresnel zone, and the far zone is the Fraunhofer zone. In pulse operation, the near zone is less irregular than in the continuous wave (CW) operation.

Ultrasound waves can be focused with lenses, mirrors, curved transducers, and electronically. Figure 7 illustrates the methods of mechanical, fixed focusing. The lenses are built of plastic materials, and the shape of a focusing lens can be convex or concave, depending on ultrasound propagation speed in the lens material. Ultrasound mirrors are built as thin structures containing air in order to obtain nearly total reflection. During the production stage, a curved transducer is formed into a focusing shape (e.g., paraboloid). All these focusing methods have a focusing distance determined by their shape, which cannot be changed. In practice, this means that there should be as many different probes as many different foci are needed. Since the focusing zones are fairly long, the number of probes at one frequency would not be more than three, usually two. Electronic focusing is illustrated in Figure 8. One can electronically focus a beam only if the transducer is composed of separate elements, which can be separately activated, and which can separately receive signals from the body. In our example, the composite transducer consists of three rings,

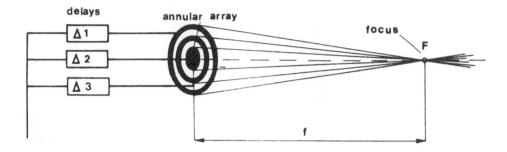

FIGURE 8.   An anular array consists of anuli of piezoelectric material that can be activated separately. The focus of such a composite transducer can be adjusted by changing the delays. Larger delays between activations yield a nearer focus.

one within another. If we define a focus depth (f) along the transducer axis, we can see that the distances from different rings to the focus point (F) are different, so that ultrasound pulses need different times to reach F. If we now transmit from the outermost ring first, then from the second ring, and after another delay from the central transducer, with the delays in activation adjusted so that they compensate for the different travel times, then the ultrasound pulses from all the three rings meet at the same time at point F. This in fact is focusing. The distance f depends on the delays and can be chosen by outside controls. Therefore, such a focusing system is flexible with a broad choice of focusing depths.

So far, we have spoken about focusing transmission. Reception focusing follows basically the same rules. In fixed focusing transducers, the transmission and the reception characteristics are equal and the round trip focusing is a result of both. In electronic focusing, these two can be made different, in fact, one can make the receiving focus follow the ultrasound pulse as it transverses the body, thus making a nearly continuous "dynamic" focus.

Lately, a mathematical method for improving the resolving power of echoscopes, previously used only in military applications, has been implemented in medical echoscopes. This computed echography is based on the fact that if the response of a system on the simplest reflector is known and sufficient computer power is provided, one can untangle the effects of the beam shape from the real characteristics of the imaged object.

Properties of the ultrasound beam are very complicated; we mentioned only the most important and those that are of greater practical importance to the user of modern scanners. Other characteristics of the beam such as sidelobes (auxiliary beams) and quantitative evaluation of beam properties can be found in more detailed and dedicated literature.

So far we have spoken only of the distribution in space, but the time distribution, the pulses, deserve mention too. The pulses sent out from the transducer are short, usually 2 to 4 cycles long. This means that for higher frequencies, the pulses can be made shorter, with a consequence of a better depth (axial) resolving power. The actual length of such pulses is about 1 μs (1 millionth of a second). This means that when defining the intensity of ultrasound, one must clearly state whether it is the average intensity or the intensity during only the pulse itself. The difference is large and of utmost importance when considering possible hazards of ultrasound. The time average intensity can be calculated by multiplying the intensity during the pulse with the ratio of "on" time (actual transmission time) to total time. If there are 1000 pulses per second and each of them has a duration of 1 μs, the ratio is 1/1000, i.e., the time average is 1 thousandth of the intensity during the pulse duration. Of course, when considering possible hazards, one must also take into account the space concentration (focusing) by taking the ratio of the surface area of the transducer and the area of the cross section at the focus. Therefore, when looking at some quoted intensity data, one must be aware of whether it is the time-average-space-average (SATA) or space-peak-time-peak (SPTP) value. Examining the matter in more detail, it turns out to be more complicated, but the above outline is the basic logic.

C. Echoscope Probes and Scanning Systems

The echoscope probe is the device containing one or more ultrasound transducers used for transmitting and receiving ultrasound. At present, the probes are built in such a manner as to automatically scan the interior of the body with which they are put in contact via some coupling agent (oil, gel). They usually operate fast enough to give a real-time image, (i.e., about 20 images per second). Occasionally, the images are composed slower with an added quality in detail resolution. The type of probe determines to a great extent the scanner properties and field of application.

Figure 9 illustrates a number of probes presently in routine use. Probe 9a is called a linear array. It contains a number of narrow, ribbon-like transducers, all of them separately connected to a cable and connector. There are usually about 64 such transducers in a probe of between 5 and 12 cm in length. Each of the transducers can have additional grooves etched to improve some of the directivity characteristics. The width of the ribbon-like transducers is too small to make a good beam, so one must activate more than one transducer at a time to obtain a composite transducer much larger than wavelength. A way to do this is to activate groups of transducers, e.g., first group 1-10, then group 2-11, then group 3-12, and so on all the way to group 55-64. In this way, one obtains a shift equal to the width of a single transducer with an apparent composite transducer ten single widths wide. Furthermore, the shifting is the actual scanning of the area in front of the probe, without any mechanical movement. In addition to the shifting-scanning, one adds delays to activation of single transducers in a group obtaining electronic focusing as previously explained for the composite ring transducer. Of course this electronic focusing applies to only one plane. In the other plane, there is a fixed focus lens. This type of transducer is used mainly in obstetrics, breast, and thyroid scanning.

Figure 9d and c illustrates the most commonly used mechanical sector scanners. They produce an approximately triangular image. In both types, the transducers are mechanically moved, thereby scanning the area in front of them. The probe illustrated in Figure 9d is a rocking probe, i.e., a transducer that is made to rock in front of an acoustical window in order to scan whatever is in front of the window. The rocking movement is not smooth but rather stepwise, and the probe spends at each increment angle the time needed for the transmission-reception sequence.

The probe illustrated in Figure 9c contains three to five transducers mounted on a turning wheel. Each of the transducers is activated and used only at the time when it traverses in front of the acoustic window. This movement is stepwise too, and the data are gathered along predefined lines with each of the transducers. In fact, the images obtained with the different transducers overlap. The property of the sector transducers is that they have a small acoustic window and can look to the side. Therefore, they are applied for gynecology, the upper abdomen, and cardiology.

The probe illustrated in Figure 9e uses an anular array for focusing and an ultrasonic mirror for scanning. The ultrasound pulses are transmitted onto the mirror and the echoes return to the anular array transducer via the mirror. The mirror itself is tilting, thereby sending the beam in different directions within the body.

The probe illustrated in Figure 9b is called a curvilinear probe (sometimes called a convex probe) and is basically built and activated like the linear array, but yielding an image format between the rectangular (like the linear array) and sector format. The image looks like a trapezoid.

The phased array illustrated in Figure 9f has the transducers mounted in an array like the linear array, but it is much shorter (1 to 2 cm). In this case, both the focusing and the beam

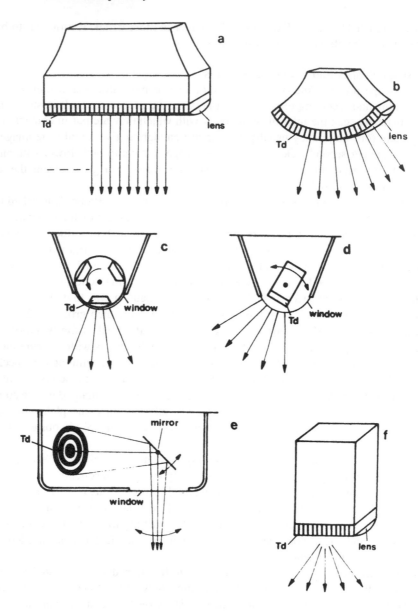

FIGURE 9.   Real-time probe types. (a) A linear array of transducers (td). Square image
format. (b) A curvilenear probe. A trapezoid image and an acoustic window of dimensions
between the linear and sector probes. (c) A rotating mechanical sector. Sector image and
small acoustic window. (d) A rocking mechanical sector probe. Sector image and small
acoustic window.(e) An anular array for focusing and an ultrasonic mirror for scanning
mounted in a housing yield high-quality sector images. (f) A phased array uses electronic
delays for both steering and focusing of the beam.

steering (change of its angle) are achieved with different delays in activation of the arrayed
transducers. The probe produces a sector image without the use of moving parts. For a long
time this system was very esteemed in echocardiography, but was less used in the upper
abdomen due to its problems with beam sidelobes. At present, the problem of sidelobes has
been solved to a great extent in the higher class instruments.

The probes as described are the most common types used in transcutaneous contact
scanning. There is a large variety of ways of combining these principles and adjustments
for specific uses.

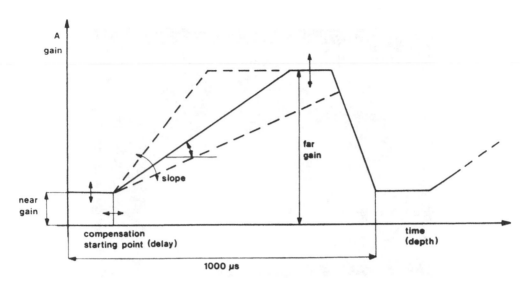

FIGURE 10. An illustration of the TGC amplifier gain variation. The near, the far, and the overall gain can be changed. The compensation slope can be adjusted and so can the compensation starting point (delay).

For ophthalmology and breast scanning, one often uses built-in waterbath probes and water transducers. Special probes for intraoperative use, for transvaginal, transvesical, or transrectal scanning have been developed. Transesophageal probes for echocardiography have been developed. Special attachments or holes in the probes for puncture needle guidance have been developed in order to keep the needle within the scanning plane under a predefined angle. All these are adaptations of the above mentioned principles to specific and special needs. To describe them all would require many printed pages, but they can all be understood if the basic principles are clear.

D. Attenuation Compensation: TGC

We have already mentioned the TGC system that is used for compensation of ultrasound attenuation in tissues. Echoes that return from deeper reflectors must be amplified more because they have been more absorbed and scattered under way. The echoes from deeper structures come later and so the TGC system compensates the attenuation by amplifying more the echoes that come later. The gain changes from minimum to maximum during each transmission-reception cycle (i.e., 1000 times per second or so). Figure 10 is a graphical representation of gain change during one cycle. The actual attenuation follows an exponential law and so does the TGC amplifier — with the opposite sign. The graphical representation in Figure 10 shows the increase of gain as linear for simplicity. Basically, one can by separate controls change the initial gain, the gain slope, the far gain, and the compensation starting point. In more attenuating tissues, the compensation slope must be steeper. The TGC system thus changes the relative amplifications at different depths. One can, with a separate control, change the overall gain, i.e., push up or lower the whole gain curve in Figure 10. In Figure 11, some examples of adjustment and misadjustment of the TGC system are shown.

There are some systems that have a present TGC function and then a set of sliding controls for modification of the TGC curve to particular needs and at different depths.

E. Dynamic Range

When speaking about the dynamic range of bright dots seen on a TV screen, we mean the ratio of brightnesses of the brightest and the least bright spot still visible on the screen. If we speak of the dynamic range of echo intensities of interest, we mean the ratio of the

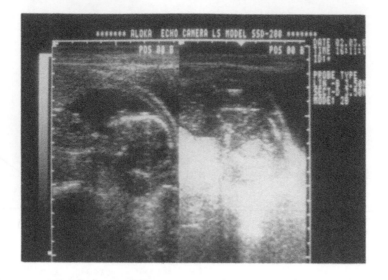

A

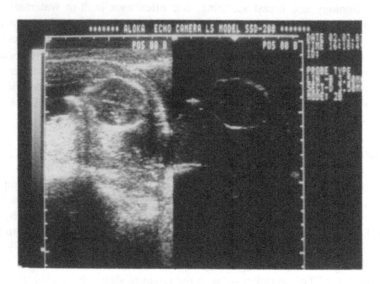

B

FIGURE 11. (A) On the left side of the figure, there is an example of optimal amplification of echoes. On the right side, misadjustment of the TCG system is illustrated as too high amplification of deep echoes. (B) An example of optimal TCG adjustment (left) compared to too low overall gain (right). (C) Too high amplification of superficial echoes (right) compared to well-adjusted image (left).

largest and the smallest echo still interesting for our purpose. When speaking about the dynamic range of our amplifier, we mean the ratio of the largest and the smallest signal which can still correctly be amplified without being cut off or saturated. A broad dynamic range of gray-scale representation of echoes on the display means that we shall see the very large and the very small echoes represented at the same time in the same image with different shades of gray. The image is ''soft''. A narrow dynamic range of echoes representation on

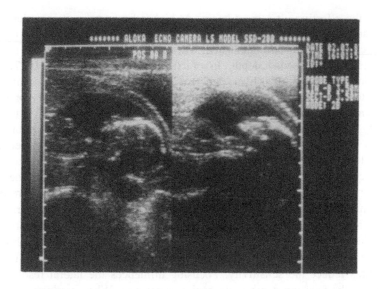

FIGURE 11C.

a gray-scale display means that there will be fewer gray tones at our disposal for representing different echo intensities; the image is "hard". For general examination where we wish to get some information on everything in the scanner field of view, a broad dynamic range is useful. If we wish to measure precisely only the most prominent structures like bones of a fetus, a lower dynamic and lower sensitivity image are more useful.

The actual range of echo intensities of interest is extremely large and many of the processes in echography are connected in series, like attenuation and amplification. This means that when dealing with actual values, we have to multiply large numbers and a large range of numbers. On the other hand, human senses like vision and hearing have quasilogarithmic characteristics so that expressing values of gain, attenuation, brightness, and dynamics is more practical and natural in a logarithmic measure — the decibel (dB). The decibel difference of two intensities is described by the following equation:

$$R_I = 10 \log \frac{I_2}{I_1}$$

Tables of ratios corresponding to decibel differences can be found in textbooks and manuals. It is important to note that a difference in decibel means the ratio — not the absolute value. Strictly speaking, only intensities, energies, and similar "squared" values should be expressed in decibels. Linear values like pressure, voltage, and absolute velocities should be expressed in nepers, another logarithmic measure; however, in actual scanners, these values are often expressed in decibels as well, only defined as follows:

$$R_P = 20 \log \frac{P_2}{P_1}$$

F. Some Notes on Resolution and Practical Use

An essential parameter in the quality and accuracy of ultrasound diagnostics is the resolution. The resolution of an echoscope can be defined as the smallest distance of two reflectors at which the reflectors can still be resolved as separate entities. Resolution can be divided into lateral and axial (depth) resolution. The lateral resolution depends basically on the width of the effective ultrasound beam. At higher frequencies it is easier to achieve a narrower beam (shorter wavelength!), but for deeper structures, one has to use lower frequencies, because they are less attenuated. Therefore, one uses the highest frequency that still can penetrate the needed depth. In practice, this means that in 1987, for general abdominal diagnostics in adults (liver, pancreas, pelvic tumors), one uses central frequency probes of 3 to 3.5 MHz; for children scanning, neonatal scanning, early pregnancy, and thin adult gynecological patients, 3.5 to 5 MHz; and for breast and neck, 5 to 10 MHz.

As already mentioned, the lateral resolution depends on the effective beam width; i.e., on the beam width, where there is sufficient ultrasound intensity to register at a certain sensitivity setting the echoes from the reflectors of interest. Reducing the sensitivity of our scanner (by reducing the transmitted ultrasound intensity or the overall gain) means reducing the effective beam width, but at the same time it means loosing the weakest reflectors from the image. Therefore, the resolution is not equal for differently strong reflectors in an image. In practice, inspect with a good resolution the strong and the weak reflectors in the same image at different sensitivity settings. When looking at pregnancy, one should gain an overview of the fetus at a higher sensitivity and dynamics, and then when measuring the bony structures reduce the sensitivity. Focusing influences the lateral resolution, so it is useful to adjust the focusing depth to the region of interest. When working with fixed focus probes, the correct probe must be chosen, e.g., for neonatal brain, a focus depth of 4 cm, and for liver examination, 8 cm.

The axial resolution is at present always better than the lateral. The depth resolution depends on the quality of echo return time registration and this can be achieved better than focusing the beam. Therefore, if we wish to image a thin blood vessel, we should use the depth resolution, i.e., orientate the probe so that the vessel lies perpendicular to the scanning beam. In the image, the blood vessel will then lie horizontally. Resolution of objects in the image depends on the contrast of the structures to be seen to their surroundings. For example, in the breast one can easily find cysts of 3 to 4 mm (at 5 MHz), while it may be hard to recognize a solid tumour of 8 to 9 mm. Apart from diagnosing by recognition of a structure, one often measures some dimensions like the skull or bones of the fetus. The results are compared with standard, normal tables. It is of utmost importance to measure the dimensions in the same way as was done when gathering normal data. Using normal graphs or tables without knowing how they have been measured means counting on pure luck.

Operator's fatigue influences the measurement accuracy. After examining 30 patients, an average operator should have a good rest or else the measurement errors become unacceptable.

G. Looking at the Image, Artifacts

At present, the majority of instruments uses only the information about the maximum amplitude of an echo. Data such as frequency spectrum, phase, or scattering angle distribution are lost. Still, the interference patterns obtained from parenchymatose organs can be recognized as normal or abnormal in many instances. Such a qualitative characterization depends on clinical experience and it is done relative to surrounding tissues. A small part of a liver parenchyma image could easily be mistaken for the placenta or kidney parenchyma without additional data.

Lately, a lot of work has been put into more exact characterization of tissues. Different investigators are trying, with initial success, to use measured data on echo spectrum modification, attenuation coefficient, and velocity for a quantitative approach. Histograms of echo amplitude distribution within an area within an image can be made in some commercial scanners. There are realistic chances for these investigations to yield quantitative characterization data in the not too distant future. A mathematically less exact but indispensable kind of tissue characterization is recognition of artifacts. We shall list some of the most usual artifacts in B-scan images (Figure 12).

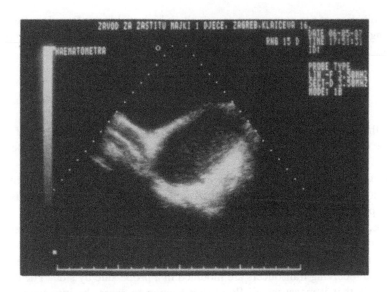

FIGURE 12. An example of increased echoes behind the cyst due to attenuation of soundwaves.

1.   Behind cysts, a zone of the increased echoes appears if the liquid in the cyst attenuates sound waves less than the surrounding tissue.
2.   Behind the lateral walls of the cysts, one can often see shadowing.
3.   Behind the bones, an ultrasonic shadow appears due to the increased attentuation in the bone. The bone image, if obtained, is grossly deformed due to a much higher ultrasound propagation speed in the bone.
4.   Behind gas bubbles in the intestines, one can see shadows, multiple reflections (reverberation), and refraction, which usually makes diagnostics under such circumstances impossible.
5.   Behind parallel layers (i.e., fatty tissue, skin muscle, etc.) one can see parallel lines or multiple images due to the reverberation of ultrasound, which is a multiple reflection of pulses back and forth between the layers.
6.   Adult skull introduces so much refraction that B scanning of the brain is presently not feasible.

IV. DOPPLER EFFECT AND ITS USE

If we imagine a transmitter and a receiver of ultrasound, which relatively do not move, then the receiver receives the same frequency of ultrasound, which is transmitted by the transmitter. However, if the receiver travels away from the transmitter at a velocity v, the receiver will register a lower frequency of ultrasound than the actually transmitted one. Conversely, if the transmitter and the receiver approach at the velocity v, the received frequency is higher than the transmitted one. This phenomenon is called the Doppler effect. If we direct the ultrasound beam from a transmitter-receiver probe onto a flow of erythrocytes, the reflected wave frequency is higher if the blood flows toward the probe and lower if it flows away. By measuring the difference in the transmitted and the received frequency (the Doppler shift), we can determine the velocity of blood flow. The Doppler shift is proportional to the component of the blood velocity along the ultrasound beam. If the angle between the beam and the flow is 90°, the velocity is equal to zero and we cannot use the Doppler effect for the measurement.

For determination of the component of velocity which yields the Doppler effect, we must know the angle between the flow to be measured and the ultrasound beam. Knowing this, we can calculate the flow velocity by the following formula:

$$\Delta f = \frac{2f_t \, v \, \cos\alpha}{c}$$

where Δf is the Doppler shift, f_t is the transmitted frequency, v is the velocity of erythrocyte movement, c is the ultrasound propagation speed, and α is the angle between the ultrasound beam and the flow direction.

In real measurements of blood flow, there is always a full spectrum of different velocities within any blood vessel and the average velocity, if needed, can be calculated using a built-in microcomputer.

In practice, Doppler systems with CW transmission and systems with pulses — pulsed Doppler — are applied. The CW systems transmit and receive ultrasound waves continually and measure the Doppler shift between the transmitted and the received wave. The transmitting and the receiving transducers are mounted in a probe side by side. The disadvantage of this sytem is that it measures all flows that happen to cross the ultrasound beam — it has no depth resolution. On the other hand, very high velocities present no problem for the CW Doppler. The pulsed Doppler system measures the Doppler shift on the echoes of short ultrasound pulses transmitted into the body. By choosing the delay between transmission and reception, we can choose the depth at which to measure the blood flow. Therefore, we can choose one single blood vessel at a known depth in which to measure the flow. Thus, this system has a depth resolution. Its disadvantage is that it cannot measure as high a velocity as the CW Doppler, because the pulsed Doppler does not "look" at the vessel all the time, but takes a limited number of samples in time.

Due to the outlined limitations, combinations of the two systems are sometimes used (e.g., in echocardiography). In practice, it is sometimes hard to find the blood vessel of interest blindly, and therefore, systems are built to combine a B-mode real-time scanner and a Doppler velocity measurement system. One finds the blood vessel of interest on the two-dimensional image and aims with the Doppler instrument at the flow. The flow spectrum as shown in Figure 13 is a quantitative method of showing the flow, but sometimes one would obtain enough clinical information from just seeing a qualitative two-dimensional map of flows in an area. For this purpose, the color-coded flow mapping systems have been developed (sometimes called "color Doppler") which fill into a two-dimensional gray-scale image the flows in a color code. If one is interested in quantitative data from some point in the color-coded flow map, it must still be measured in one of the previously mentioned ways. In evaluating a flow, one takes into account not only the frequency (velocity) spectrum at some moment, but the whole time variation of the flow. Proper use of sophisticated Doppler systems requires an additional education similar to what is needed for 2D echography.

V. SOME PRACTICAL ADVICE

1.   The skin must be oiled or some contact gel must be used in order to eliminate air bubbles between the probe and the skin.
2.   The overview scan must be made with a broad dynamic range (40 dB or more) and sufficient sensitivity.
3.   For measurement of fetal head and bones or to obtain clearer edges of structures, the dynamic range should be reduced, as well as the overall sensitivity. In simpler instruments there might not be a dynamic range control, in which case one can only use

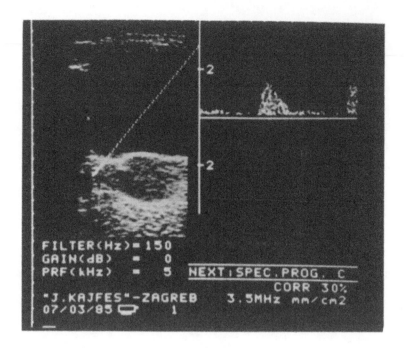

FIGURE 13. An example of the Doppler flow spectrum obtained from the ovarian artery.

the overall sensitvity control that is sufficient for bone measurement, but not for edge enhancement.

4. The echo density at all depths should be equal for similar structures. This is controlled by the TGC controls.

5. The caliper crosses, asterisks, etc., must always be placed in the same way in order to obtain reproducible measurements.

6. Frequency and focus distance of the probe must correspond to the actual requirements. Maximum frequency compatible with penetration power must be used.

7. If a puncture is guided by ultrasound, one must take care to keep the whole needle within the scanning plane, i.e., within the section thickness.

8. When purchasing a scanner, one must take into account how well the future operator is educated. The most sophisticated scanners can cost ten times as much as a middle-class instrument, but its advantages can be put in use only by an expert.

9. When scanning superficial organs (breast, thyroid), a delay layer must be interpolated between the probe and the skin in the form of a water layer or a special nonliquid gel.

REFERENCES

1. **Wells, P. N. T.,** *Biomedical Ultrasonics,* Academic Press, New York, 1977.
2. **Woodcock, J. P.,** *Ultrasonics,* Adam Hilger, Bristol, 1979.
3. **Seto, W. W.,** *Acoustics,* McGraw-Hill, New York, 1971.
4. **Kremkau, F. W.,** *Diagnostic Ultrasound,* Grune & Stratton, New York, 1984.
5. The Bioeffects Committee of the AIUM Safety Considerations for Diagnostic Ultrasound, *Am. Int. Ultrasound. Med.,* Publications, Bethesda, MD, 1984.
6. The Watchdog Group of the European Federation of Societies for Ultrasound in Medicine and Biology, *Eur. Med. Ultrasonics,* 6, 8, 1984.

Chapter 2

PRINCIPLES OF PATHOPHYSIOLOGY OF INFERTILITY ASSESSMENT AND TREATMENT*

Joseph G. Schenker, Aby Lewin, and Menashe Ben-David

TABLE OF CONTENTS

* The authors of this chapter have decided that references are unnecessary.

I. INTRODUCTION

Infertility has been defined as failure to conceive within 1 year of unprotected coitus. Primary infertility refers to couples who had never achieved conception. Secondary infertility may follow one or more previous conceptions.

Infertility is regarded as one of the main problems of the human race. The Ebers papyres contain many detailed recipes for restoration of childbearing. The aspects of procreation are emphasized in Judeo-Christian tradition. Therefore, in the Bible, both the Old and New Testament refer broadly to the question of infertile and sterile couples. The different aspects of infertility are prominantly mentioned in the Hypocratic, Galenic, and Middle Age medical writings. The importance adhered to avoiding sterility exists in most societies that developed beliefs about how to cure infertility. Infertility is not a medical problem of a female or male partner; it is a pathological condition of a couple. Failure to conceive may be tragic for some couples: it can result in marital crisis, unhappiness, and psychosomatic health problems.

The prevalence of infertility varies in different parts of the world and it even varies among the different ethnic groups and regions in the same country. It is estimated that 10 to 15% of couples in the Western Hemisphere are infertile, which makes infertility one of the most common problems for which people seek medical care. Infertility is also reported to be very common in Africa and in certain Asian countries. In North America and Western Europe, the prevalence of infertility is believed to have increased in the last decades as a result of delayed childbearing among couples and an increase of sexually transmitted diseases. Reproductive failure occurs as a result of anatomical, physiological, endocrinological, pathological, immunological, and psychological factors. The distribution of etiological factors in infertile couples varies among different centers all over the world.

Fertility is maximal in females around the age of 24 years, after which it gradually decreases to the age of 35, and rapidly declines thereafter. The main factor in the decline in fecundability in the 10 to 15 years before ovarian failure occurs at menopause is due to an increase in the incidence of anovulatory cycles and early pregnancy loss.

Regarding the male partner, fecundability is maximal around the age of 24 to 30 years. The biological influence of paternal age in the decline of infertility is mainly due to the decline of his sexual activity in terms of the number of ejaculations per week and the time it takes to achieve erection. Some studies have found that advanced paternal age may cause an increase in the incidence of pregnancy loss mainly due to chromosomal aberrations. Several environmental factors like nutritional disturbances, stress, exposure to drugs, and chemical and physical agents may contribute to infertility.

II. EVALUATION OF INFERTILITY

The following elements are essential in order for intrauterine conception to be initiated: (1) the testis — to produce an adequate quantity of viable sperm with normal morphology, motility, and property of fertilization; (2) the ovary, which releases a mature oocyte; (3) the sperm and oocytes must be able to meet at a proper time; and (4) endometrial preparation for successful embryo implantation.

Infertility may be caused by a single or multiple etiological factor(s). It is customary to classify the causes of infertility into the following major groups:

1. Failure of ovulation
2. Mechanical factors: including tubal pathology and peritoneal causes that disturb the ovum pick-up mechanism, transport of gametes, fertilization, and early preembryo transport
3. Uterine factors: Muellerian duct abnormalities, intrauterine adhesions and uterine tumors
4. Cervical factors: cervical anomalies and impaired cervical mucus secretion
5. Male factors: inadequate or abnormal production, ejaculation, and deposition of spermatozoa
6. Emotional aspects and sexual disturbances
7. Immunological factors
8. Unexplained infertility
9. Multifunctional factors

Medically, infertility is a rather unique condition in that one must consider two individuals. Both partners may have factors contributing to the condition of reproductive failure, therefore both must cooperate in the investigation and should be diagnosed and treated as one unit. It is generally impossible to make an etiological diagnosis of infertility at the first visit. The investigation should begin with a careful medical history and physical examination, which will exclude major medical or gynecological conditions (Figure 1). Subsequent investigations of both partners must be very specific and include tests of factors concerning fertilization and implantation.

III. UTERINE FACTOR OF INFERTILITY (FIGURES 2 AND 3)

The uterus has many significant roles in conception, implantation, and maintenance of conception. Uterine abnormalities directly responsible for infertility are congenital anomalies, myomatous tumors, intrauterine adhesions, endometritis, and adenomyosis. Congenital malformations of the uterus occur in 0.1 to 0.4% of all women. Most of the congenital uterine anomalies are due to some degree of failure of fusion or canalization of the Muellerian duct. More than 80% of women should have no difficulties in conceiving (except in cases of agenesis of uterus), although only $1/3$ will deliver a viable child because of a high rate of early and late abortions, and premature deliveries. Defects such as septate and bicornuate uterus, which are associated with the highest pregnancy loss, may be surgically corrected by metroplastic procedures.

Uterine myoma may be a cause of secondary, as well as primary, infertility. The mechanism by which myoma interferes with conception is not definitely known:

1. A submucus fibroid bulging into the cavity of the uterus may prevet fertilization or implantation by the same way as an intrauterine device.
2. The endometrium that covers the fibroid may ulcerate, become infected, and prevent a normal implantation.

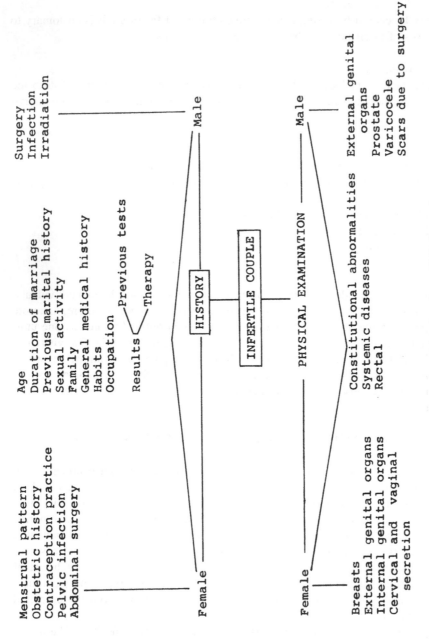

FIGURE 1.   Clinical work-up of infertile couple.

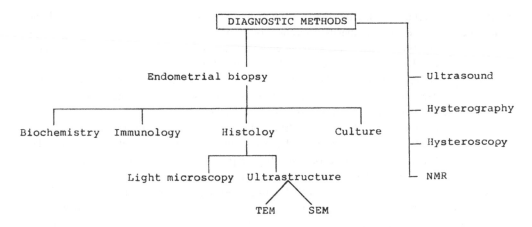

FIGURE 2.   Assessment of uterine factors of infertility.

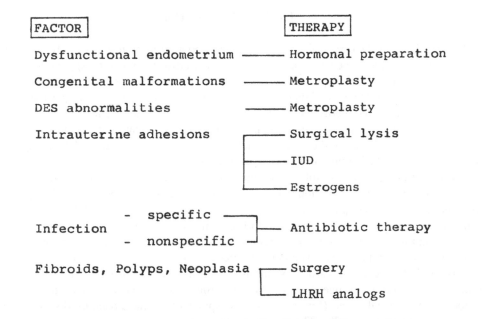

FIGURE 3.   Therapeutic approach to uterine causes of infertility.

3.   A large myoma may be a mechanical factor of infertility by constriction of tubal lumen or cause malposition of ovaries in relation to the tubal fimbria.

4.   Growth of fibroid may cause changes in the blood supply to the uterus which may prevent implantation or cause early abortions.

The most practical treatment for leiomyoma associated with infertility has been surgical removal of the tumor. Surgery is not always a satisfactory solution; it can sometimes create new problems such as formation of adhesions leading to mechanical infertility.

The use of gonadotropin-releasing hormone (Gn-RH) agonists is a new therapeutic approach. The antigonadotrophic action of luteinizing hormone-releasing hormone (LH-RH) agonists can induce regulation of fibroids by reducing follicle-stimulating hormone (FSH)-induced estrogen secretion and depriving the myoma of its growth stimulus.

Intrauterine adhesions (Asherman's syndrome) may be a cause of infertility. It is generally accompanied by menstrual disorders, mainly amenorrhea or hypomenorrhea. The cause of

infertility is uncertain. It may be due to a mechanical obstruction of the cervical canal and/
or uterine cavity, impeding sperm migration or implantation. Adhesions also may cause
defective endometrial function, an unstable endometrial environment not suitable to nidation
of the blastocyst. Diagnosis and location of intrauterine adhesions are based essentially on
hysterography and hysteroscopy. The treatment consists of surgically removing the adhesions
and at the same time preventing formation of new ones by immediate insertion of an
intrauterine device (IUD) combined with estrogen therapy.

Inflammatory diseases of the endometrium, both specific and nonspecific, are known
causes of infertility. Tuberculosis (TB) of the endometrium, which is always a secondary
infection, is still a common cause of infertility, especially in many developing countries.
The end result of TB endometritis is severe intrauterine adhesions, often with total atresia
of the uterine cavity, leading to sterility. Inflammatory changes and immunological factors
present in the endometrium and in the uterine secretion are among the potential hazards for
blastocyst implantation. Our present knowledge on the function of the endometrium is
limited.

IV. CERVICAL FACTOR

Abnormalities of the cervix and its secretion are reported to be responsible for infertility
in 5 to 10% of couples. The term "cervical factor in infertility" should be applied to couples
in whom the male is normospermic, but repeated postcoital tests are negative. The cervix
seems to be an important part of successful fertilization. It contributes to the sperm transport
from the vagina to the uterus and to the process of capacitation. The cervical factor of
infertility may be considered a two-component problem: an anatomical and/or functional
defect. Congenital defects of the cervix, resulting from *in utero* exposure to DES, may result
in infertility by reducing the number of sperm transmitted through the cervical canal. Anatomical conditions such as isolated absence of cervix (a rare congenital malformation),
stenosis of cervix, prolapse or elongation, malposition, and status of postcervical amputation
may interfere with conception. Cervical trauma, resulting in extreme dilatation, conization,
cautery, or cryosurgery, may contribute to impair mucus secretion.

The main function of the cervix is secretion of mucus by the nonciliated columnar epithelial
cells lining the cervical canal. The cervical mucus has biochemical and biophysical characteristics that have cyclic variations during a menstrual cycle. The secretion of cervical
mucus is stimulated by estrogens and inhibited by progesterone. Cyclic changes in rheological
properties of cervical mucus (ferning, viscosity, spinnbarkeit) have been used in an attempt
to predict ovulation clinically. The mucus has two apparently opposing functions: a barrier
preventing the entrance of a hostile vaginal environment like bacteria, secretion of low pH
into the uterus, and, on the other hand, allowing the passage of sperm at the preovulatory
period. The biological valve action of the cervix is dependent on the rheological properties
of the mucus.

The main functions of the cervix and its secretion in the conception process are

1.   Facilitating sperm passage from the vagina into the uterus at ovulation
2.   Protecting sperm from the hostile environment of the vagina and of its phagocytosis
3.   Supplementing the energy requirement of the sperm
4.   Acting as a sperm reservoir
5.   Providing a site for sperm capacitation

The mechanism of cervical mucus production and its effect on sperm mucus interaction
are still unclear.

Evaluation of cervical factor and sperm cervical mucus interaction may be difficult due to multiplicity of etiology (Figure 4). Postcoital examination of cervical mucus is a basic test for evaluation of the infertile couple. It should be initiated before more invasive procedures are employed. Semen analysis and examination of the five important properties of cervical mucus (amount, viscosity, ferning, spinnbarkeit, and cellularity) should precede postcoital tests. Culture of endocervical mucus should determine the presence and type of infection. In cases of repeated abnormal postcoital tests, there is an indication for the *in vitro* cervical mucus sperm penetration test. The treatment of cervical factor depends on the etiology of the condition (Figure 4). The presence of hostile mucus at the ovulatory period of the cycle probably should be evaluated for anovulation and treated with gonadotropin preparations. If cervical infection is present, a broad spectrum of antibiotics may be applied. In cases of pathological lesions and of disturbances of sperm deposition, surgical management should be applied and/or intrauterine insemination.

In patients with cervical factor of infertility who did not respond to conventional techniques of therapy, *in vitro* fertilization, embryo transfer, and especially a gamete intrafallopian transfer (GIFT) procedure may be tried.

V. INFERTILITY DUE TO OVULATORY FACTORS

A. Neuroendocrine Regulation of Infertility

1. The Hypothalamus

Fertility is a biological function regulated by an integrative neuroendocrine mechanism primarily located in the hypothalamus. Schally was the first to isolate the hypothalamic hormone LH-RH (Gn-RH) that controls the synthesis and release of the pituitary LH and FSH, and succeeded to synthesize it.

Gn-RH is secreted by neuroendocrine cells located in the arcuate-located nucleus of the hypothalamus. It arrives to the interior pituitary via the hypophysical portal blood system. Despite the fact that Gn-RH can be synthesized independently in the hypothalamus, its synthesis degree and especially the timing of its release are highly dependent on stimuli originated in various parts of the central nervous system (CNS), particularly the limbic system. Various neurotransmitters, mainly noradrenaline, dopamine, and 5-hydroxytryptamine (serotonin), can effect the secretion of Gn-RH in the hypothalamus. Other less influential neurotransmitters such as histamine, glutamic acid, melatonin, β-endorphins, and enkephalins also may indirectly participate in the regulation of Gn-RH secretion. Thus, extroceptive stimuli such as stress, which may activate some of the above neurotransmitters, may eventually alter the gonadal function. It is well known that blindness, deafness, and stress are often associated with precocious or delayed sexual maturation.

Knobil observed that pulsatile secretion of Gn-RH is necessary to stimulate pituitary gonadotropin and to initiate and sustain ovulatory menstrual cycles in primates. An alteration in the pulsatile secretion of Gn-RH will cause an abnormality or cessation of the reproductive function.

2. The Pituitary

The adenohypophysis is an intermediate member in a dynamic relationship between the hypothalamus and the peripheral gonadal glands. The adenohypophysis modulates the function of both the gonads and the hypothalamus via a "short loop" mechanism. In turn, the pituitary is affected by hormonal signals from both the hypothalamus and the peripheral gonads. The pituitary is affected not only by the hypothalamic Gn-RH, but also by the hypothalamic dopamine, which in turn regulate the synthesis and release of FSH, LH, and prolactin, each of which can affect gonadal function.

The pituitary gonadotropes possess specific binding sites (receptors) to Gn-RH. The binding of Gn-RH to the pituitary plasma membrane receptor appears to involve amino acids in positions 1 and 10 which are in close physical proximity at the lowest energy state of the molecule. However, the first three amino acids are required for an ultimate functional effect of gonadotropin secretion. While the procedure of binding of Gn-RH to its pituitary receptor does not need the presence of calcium ions, it is well established that ionic calcium (Ca^{2+}) acts as a second messenger for Gn-RH, namely the transfer of the hormone-receptor signal into the cell.

3. The Ovaries

Most of the abundant developing primordial follicles in the ovaries undergo atresia unless they receive stimulation by the pituitary gonadotropin FSH. The rise in plasma FSH observed in the waning days of the previous luteal phase and at the beginning of the menstrual cycle activates and prevents atresia of some of the developing primordial follicles. The first follicle able to respond to FSH stimulation may achieve an early lead that it never relinquishes. Thus, once growth is initiated, the granulosa cells undergo proliferation and the theca layer begins to organize from the surrounding stroma. Steroidogenesis also is stimulated by action of FSH. Granulosa cells can synthesize all three steroids progestins, androgens, and estrogens. The conversion of androgens to estrogens is induced by the aromatizing enzymes, which are induced by action of FSH. Another action of FSH is that in conjunction with estradiol there is stimulation of synthesis of further receptors of FSH. Such synergistic action of FSH and estradiol can be achieved both *in vivo* and *in vitro*. Under this synergistic action of estradiol and FSH, there is an increase of follicular fluid production and accumulation and formation of antral follicle.

In normal folliculogenesis, FSH is detectable in the follicular fluid and the concentration of estrogens in the antral fluid exceeds that of androgens. When FSH is not detectable in the follicular fluid, then androgens predominate and further follicular development may cease.

In later antral development, there is interaction between thecal and granulosa compartments. At the beginning, LH receptors are present only in the thecal cells and FSH receptors only in the granulosa cells. In response to LH, thecal tissue is stimulated to secrete androgens that later can be converted through FSH-induced aromatization to estrogens in the granulosa cells. The successful conversion of androgens to estrogens, which in turn may increase FSH receptors, will lead to enhancement of local concentration of FSH and ensure further mitosis and follicular development. This will end with "selection" of the predominant follicle to reach full maturation and ovulation, while other follicles will "suffer" from the decline or circulating FSH that takes place due to the negative action of the increasing amounts of estrogen or the hypothalamic-pituitary-gonadotropin axis. If for any reason there is an interference with the aromatase activity at the gonadal level (e.g., by high levels of prolactin) and/or the concentration of androgens exceeds that of estrogens, follicular maturation may be inhibited.

Further follicular development takes place in the leading follicle when LH receptors on the granulosa cell membranes are being synthesized. Presence of both FSH and estradiol is essential for the synthesis of LH receptors in the granulosa cells. Such conditions exist only in the leading follicle, which has the capacity to bind even the declined peripheral FSH concentration (due to high receptor levels) and thus to induce a microenvironment rich with estradiol. Increasing amount of peripheral estradiol can act directly on the pituitary gonadotropes to trigger positive feedback on LH. Concentrations higher than 200 pg/ml of estradiol are needed to achieve the positive feedback on pituitary LH. Moreover, estrogen feedback on LH secretion enhances not only the quantity of LH release, but also its quality by modulation of the LH molecule to one with a higher biological activity. During the late follicular phase, estrogens rise rapidly, reaching a maximum 24 to 36 h before the ovulation. Concomitantly, there is a decline in the circulating FSH to this nadir while FSH increases

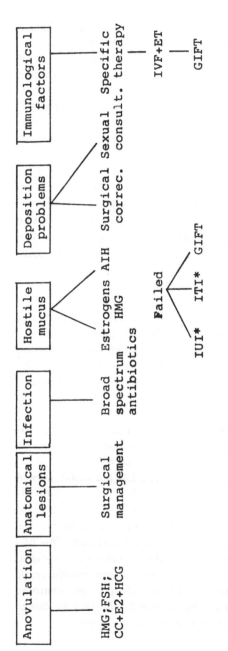

FIGURE 4. Etiology and therapy in cases of severe cervical factors of infertility.

*IUI – intrauterine insemination.
*ITI – intratubal insemination.

steadily and then rapidly in a surge-like burst at midcycle, accompanied by a lesser surge of FSH. In the presence of high estradiol concentration and adequate amount of FSH, activation of the granulosa cell LH receptors by the abundant LH will lead to a process of luteinization and an increase in progesterone production. If, however, there is no adequate amounts of either estradiol or FSH in the microenvironment of the follicles, the follicles react to LH bolus with atresia rather than luteinization.

Similarly, the premature administration of human chorionic gonadotropin (HCG) to induce ovulation may disrupt further development and result in a failure of ovulation.

The process of luteinization and progesterone production is mediated by activation of adenylate cyclase in the LH-mediated process of separation of the egg cell with its surrounding granulosa-corona cells from the cumulus oophorus and paves the way for its extrusion from the follicle. Progesterone and/or LH may enhance the activity of proteolytic enzymes, resulting in digestion of collagen in the follicular wall and increasing its distensibility. Apart from that, as a result of LH increase and activation of its receptors in the follicle, prostaglandins of the F and E series increase markedly in preovulatory follicular fluid reaching a peak at ovulation. Prostaglandins play an important role in the mechanical rupture and the extrusion of the egg with its cumulus cells from the follicle. The mechanism by which prostaglandins aid the follicular rupture and egg expulsion is not fully known. However, they may enhance the activity of proteolytic enzymes and/or they may contract the smooth muscle cells found in the ovary. Inhibition of prostaglandin synthesis by indomethacin or aspirin derivatives may inhibit follicular rupture without affecting other LH-induced processes of luteinization or egg maturation.

B. Anovulation Disorders

Anovulation can be due to organic or functional disorders of the hypothalamus, pituitary, and ovary. It is often the result of a combination of factors affecting the hypothalamic-pituitary-ovarian axis. From 20 to 25% of the cases of infertility are related to anovulation. The World Health Organization (WHO) proposed a useful classification of the patients with ovulatory disturbances which rests primarily upon the level of gonadotropins, prolactin, and sex steroids (Figure 5):

1. Hypothalamic pituitary failure: anorexia nervosa, Kalmann's syndrome and the patient's present clinical symptoms of primary or secondary amenorrhea. Serum levels of FSH, LH, and estradiol are low. The levels of prolactin are normal.
2. Hypothalamic pituitary dysfunction: serum levels of FSH and LH are within normal range, but the cyclic release of gonadotropins necessary for induction of ovulation is absent. There is evidence for endogenous estrogen production, and prolactin levels are normal. This category may include females with hyperandrogenic activity. The patient may have presenting symptoms of amenorrhea and oligomenorrhea. This category may include patients with polycystic ovarian disease, amenorrhea associated with loss of weight, exercise, and stress, and patients with corpus luteum insufficiency.
3. Ovarian failure: patients in this group are amenorrheic with elevated gonadotropin levels and no evidence of estrogenic production. The ovarian failure may be due to gonadal dysgenesis, premature menopause, and resistant ovary syndrome.

Recent advances in understanding the pathophysiology of ovulation and the development of potent pharmacological agents have made it possible to induce ovulation in the majority of anovulatory females. At present, the majority of women whose infertility is caused by anovulation can be treated successfully.

1. Induction of Ovulation

There has been a significant progress in treatment of anovulation with different phar-

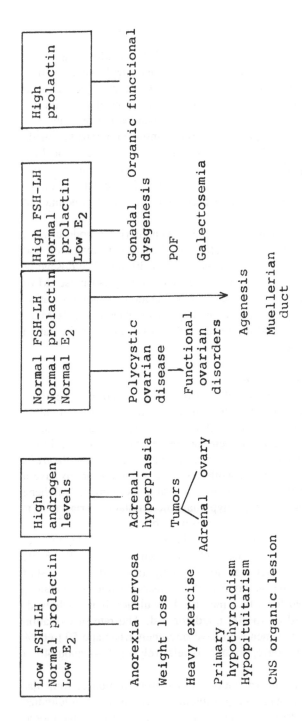

FIGURE 5. Classification of primary amenorrhea according to gonadotropin, prolactin, and sex steroid levels.

macological agents in the last 20 years. The success of therapy depends on an accurate diagnosis of underlying abnormalities responsible for anovulation and the selection of agents (one most appropriate to initiate ovulation, least expensive, and with minimum harm to the patient).

2. Induction of Ovulation with Gn-RH

Gn-RH is a decapeptide that is found in all mammalian species, including man. It is released by the hypothalamus and transported to the anterior pituitary gland, where it stimulates the release for LH and FSH. After its isolation and following Gn-RH synthesis, clinical trials were attempted with occasional success to obtain ovulation and conception with anovulatory infertility. Following more recent insight into the neuroendocrine regulation of menstruation and the development of small, automatically timed infusion pumps has made Gn-RH an effective agent for induction of ovulation. The selection of patients is critical for pulsatile administration of Gn-RH. Hypothalamic amenorrhea and hypogonadotrophic-hypogonadism constitute the main indication for Gn-RH therapy. About 200 pregnancies have been obtained. The success rate is low in amenorrheic patients with hyperprolactinemia and hyperandrogenemia.

Gn-RH may be administered by subcutaneous (s.c.) or intravenous (i.v.) mode using a computerized mini pump. The i.v. pulsatile administration resulted in high ovulation and conception rates. The usual pulse frequency recommended is every 30 min. The dosage of Gn-RH per pulse utilized for ovulation induction varies from 1 to 100 μg per pulse. Most investigators apply a dose between 1 to 20 μg per pulse. Combinations of administration of Gn-RH with other agents such as clomiphene, human menopausal gonadotropins (HMG), and HCG have been reported. Recently, Gn-RH has been used for ovarian superstimulation in the *in vitro* fertilization (IVF) programs.

3. Induction of Ovulation with Clomiphene Citrate

Clomiphene citrate (CC) is an analog of nonsteroidal estrogen (Tace) and its structure is similar to that of stilbestrol. Its biological action is to compete with estrogen for binding sites in the hypothalamus and possibly in the pituitary gland and ovary. During its administration, there is a moderate rise in FSH and LH secretion and a gradual increase in the estrogen production in the ovary. There are two isomers of clomiphene: the *cis* and the *trans* form. The *cis* form has an antiestrogenic property, while the *trans* form appears to have a mild estrogenic effect on vaginal cytology, cervical glands, and endometrium. Clomiphene therapy is indicated to patients in whom an intact hypothalamic-pituitary-ovarian axis is present. It is, therefore, the drug of choice for women who have oligomenorrhea or amenorrhea with circulatory estrogen levels in the normal range for the follicular phase of menstrual cycles. Most patients are likely to respond to clomiphene when the tonic center is still capable of producing Gn-RH — while the cyclic center is nonfunctioning. It is customary to start with a low dose of 50 mg/d for 5 d, starting on day 5 of the menstrual cycle. If ovulatory response is noted, the dose is maintained for 4 to 6 months. If ovulation is not achieved, the dosage should be gradually increased up to 200 mg/d for 5 d. The rate of ovulation achieved is in the range of 80 to 90% for women who have oligomenorrhea and 50 to 60% in patients with amenorrhea, although the conception rate is relatively small — about 40 to 45%.

The cases of conception failure are misinterpretation of ovulatory response, follicular phase defect (short or long), abnormal LH surge, corpus luteum insufficiency, and luteinize unruptured follicular syndrome. Patients treated with clomiphene are usually not monitored during the treatment cycle. Close monitoring by blood hormones measurement and ultrasonography may improve the clinical results. When ovulation occurs but there is a failure to achieve conception, one must look for other etiology of infertility, and especially the side effect of clomiphene treatment on the sperm-mucus interaction. Based on the clinical condition and the response to therapy, clomiphene might be administered concomitantly with other agents like HCG, Gn-RH, HMG, prednisone, and estrogen preparation.

4. Gonadotropin Preparations for Induction of Ovulation

Gonadotropins of human origin are obtained from postmortem pituitary glands (human pituitary gonadotropin, HPG) or human postmenopausal urine (human menopausal gonadotropin, HMG). Both are used in conjunction with HCG. The preparation most available commercially is extracted from human postmenopausal urine (pergonal). Pergonal contains both FSH and LH in a 1:1 ratio. Pure preparation of FSH is marked under the tradename of Metrodin.® The absolute indications for gonadotropin therapy are patients who lack a functioning pituitary gland either as the result of destruction by an organic lesion, or following hypophysectomy. Patients with hypothalamic-pituitary failure, women with primary or secondary amenorrhea (low levels of endogenous FSH and LH), and lack of endogenous estrogenic activity should be treated with gonadotropin therapy. Patients with anovulation associated with a variety of menstrual disorders (normal serum gonadotropin levels, estrogen activity) are suitable for treatment with gonadotropins.

Pergonal and FSH in combination with HCG is also applied in patients who have ovulated but had not conceived after 6 months of clomiphene therapy. Ovulation has occasionally been induced in patients with gonadotrophic-resistant ovary syndrome and even in rare instances in women with elevated FSH and LH levels. Recently, gonadotropin preparations in different combinations and different regimens of therapy have been used for ovarian hyperstimulation for IVF and embryo transfer (ET).

A variety of treatment schedules for gonadotropin administration for induction of ovulation have been devised. Nearly all of those schedules are based on the fact that treatment with gonadotropin preparations results specifically in follicular growth and maturation. The "variable technique" has been used more commonly; the daily dosage and duration of therapy depend on individual response. Gonadotropin preparations are very active agents for stimulating the ovary to ovulate, and with adequate therapy ovulation is achieved in 80 to 90% of the patients, although pregnancy can be expected in only 40 to 60%. The conception rate depends on the selection of patients, dose, regimen, and number of treatment cycles. Gonadotropin therapy can be applied in combination with different agents like clomiphene, Gn-RH, dexamethasone, and parlodel.

5. Complications of Induction of Ovulation

With currently available pharmacological therapy, ovulation may be successfully induced in almost every patient. However, the rate of complications is still substantial. The most common complications are ovarian hyperstimulation syndrome (OHSS), multiple gestation, and high rate of first-trimester abortions. OHSS is the most prevalent albeit the most serious complication of induction of ovulation. It is a syndrome in which induction of ovulation results in a wide spectrum of clinical and laboratory symptoms and signs: on the one end of the spectrum there is only chemical evidence of ovarian hyperstimulation with increased production of sex steroids, while on the other end of the spectrum there is a massive ovarian enlargement, ascites, pleural effusion, electrolyte imbalance, hypovolemic shock, and even thromboembolic phenomena. The incidence of OHSS varies with the different clinical conditions in which ovulation is induced, the types of preparation administered, the doses and schedules administered, and the method applied for monitoring the ovarian response.

The incidence of mild OHSS with CC is in the range of 10 to 15%. Severe OHSS with clomiphene treatment is rare. The incidence of hyperstimulation using gonadotropins is reported to be about 10% of mild grade and 0.5% of severe grade. With the induction of methods of monitoring induction of ovulation by urinary or serum estrogen estimation and the measurement of follicular growth by ultrasonography, the incidence of severe cases is decreasing.

Application of Gn-RH is associated with an OHSS rate lower than that observed during gonadotropin therapy, and is similar to that found following therapy with CC.

Multiple pregnancies is the second major complication of ovulation induction. While the rate of OHSS may be considerably reduced by careful monitoring of ovulation induction, the occurrence of multiple gestation still seems much less controllable.

The rate of multiple pregnancies with HMG-HCG is about 20 to 25%; with CC, 10%; and with Gn-RH, 7.5%.

There generally is recognized increased evidence of spontaneous abortions in the treatment of infertility and especially after induction of ovulation. The incidence of abortion after gonadotropins treatment is 25 to 30%; after CC, it is 19%; and following Gn-RH therapy, it is about 15%.

C. Prolactin and Female Infertility

The CNS exerts tonic inhibitory control on prolactin secretion. As a consequence, interference with the integrity of the normal hypothalamic-pituitary connection results in an increase in prolactin secretion. The chemical nature of the prolactin-inhibiting factor (PIF) and the possible existence of more than one PIF remain controversial. However, dopamine, a monoamine, fulfills many of the criteria of such an inhibiting factor and is considered by many workers to represent the physiologically most important PIF.

Hyperprolactinemia is today the most common pituitary disorder in men. Chronic hyperprolactinemia may result in either luteal deficiency, anovulation, oligomenorrhea, or amenorrhea with or without galactorrhea. It has been suggested that the antigonadotrophic action of hyperprolactinemia is mainly due to an activation of an inhibiting dopaminergic mechanism with the lateral palisade zone (PZ) of the medium eminence, resulting in inhibition of the secretion of LH-RH into the portal vessels.

Our early observations indicate that prolactin also exerts a direct effect on the ovaries interfering with gonadal response to exogenous gonadotropins. In addition, binding sites for prolactin were found to exist in human granulosa cells. Also, it was shown that prolactin, added to granulosa cells growing *in vitro*, may inhibit aromatase activity resulting in a decrease of estradiol synthesis and an accumulation of androgens. Thus, it is most likely that hyperprolactinemia induces infertility by acting on both levels: the hypothalamus-pituitary axis and the ovaries.

Hyperprolactinemia may result in a decrease of gonadotropin secretion and/or an inhibition of synthesis of adequate amounts of estradiol most needed within the follicular microenvironment for normal folliculogenesis and ovulation.

While a state of hypoprolactinemia may not exist (except for rare cases of pan-hypopituitarism), a condition of hyperprolactinemia is common and relatively abundant among women. The remarkable ability of the pituitary lactotropes to spontaneously and independently secrete prolactin prevents almost entirely the constitution of the hypoprolactinemic state. On the other hand, hyperprolactinemia can be easily achieved, especially in the female, due to the relatively high circulating estradiol levels. Estrogens may enhance prolactin secretion by one or both of the following ways: estrogens deliver the genetic code for prolactin synthesis and estrogens may reduce the hypothalamic dopamine availability and thereby cause prolactin hypersecretion.

In women, estradiol seems to be the principle factor causing states of transient hyperprolactinemia. In contrast to long-standing hyperprolactinemia, the transient one is brought about only after a condition of high circulating estradiol levels coupled with high lactotroph sensitivity to the estrogen is being constituted. A transitory stress state is another factor that may contribute to a condition of transient hyperprolactinemia. The most well-known causes of transient hyperprolactinemia which can induce infertility are as follows: (1) cases of preovulatory estradiol induce transient hyperprolactinemia, which may exist in normally cycling women suffering from unexplained infertility, and (2) cases of HMG provoked estradiol-induced transient hyperprolactinemia, which can lead to failure in HMG treatment (Figure 6).

Based on our clinical experience, the hyperprolactinemic state can be differentiated into two types: (1) long-standing hyperprolactinemia, which may be associated with organic lesion of the pituitary gland or functional hyperprolactinemia due to stress, postpartum, post pill, and following the use of dopamine blocker agents, or (2) transient hyperprolactinemia, which may lead to infertility by a mechanism not yet known, but which certainly differs from that of chronic hyperprolactinemia.

1. Agents that Inhibit Prolactin Secretion

The most effective prolactin-suppressing drugs are the ergot and ergolin derivatives (bromocriptine, lisuride, metergoline), which seem to act by the virtue of their dopaminergic properties. Bromocriptine (Parlodel), a dopamine agonist, is used for induction of ovulation in cases of anovulation due to hyperprolactinemia. It has two sites of action: at the level of the CNS and at the level of the pituitary gland. In a therapeutic dose of 2.5 to 7.5 mg daily, it produces rapid and prolonged inhibition of prolactin secretion. Most patients with infertility due to hyperprolactinemia respond to treatment with bromocriptine, and the great majority who conceive do so within six ovulatory cycles.

Apart from reducing prolactin secretion and release, bromocriptine also diminishes DNA synthesis and reduces mitotic activity in the pituitary tumor cells. Long-term treatment with bromocriptine in some patients with micro- or macroadenoma could reduce the volume of the tumor to the point of complete disappearance, Bromocriptine is effective in cases of transient hyperprolactinemia. It may be administered concomitantly with other agents like gonadotropin preparations and CC for induction of ovulation. The side effects of bromocriptine are hypotension, nausea, and vomiting due to the potent dopaminergic agonistic effect, especially in sensitive patients. It has been documented that induction of ovulation with bromocriptine is not associated with an increased rate of multiple gestation, abortions, or congenital malformations.

2. Ovarian Failure

Until recently, women with ovarian failure suffering primary or secondary amenorrhea, hypergonadotrophism, and hypoestrinism were considered incurably sterile. Primary ovarian failure is due to gonadal dysgenesis, Turner's syndrome, Turner-like mosaics, and in cases of mixed gonadal dysgenesis. Premature ovarian failure is a rare entity. Its incidence is 3.1% of all women. It is defined as ovarian failure characterized by secondary amenorrhea with elevated gonadotropin levels occurring prior to the age of 35 years. Premature ovarian failure may be due to premature menopause, resistant ovary syndrome, autoimmune disorders, galactosemia, ovarian destruction following surgery, radiation, and chemotherapy.

Since the introduction of oocyte donation with the IVF and ET program, 69 pregnancies and 45 births were reported in patients with ovarian failure.

VI. MALE INFERTILITY

The contribution of male factor to infertility is about 30 to 40%. In the last 20 years, significant advances have been made in the understanding of many aspects of normal male reproductive functions, but the pathogenesis of the majority of disorders resulting in infertility remains obscure and the effectiveness of the different modalities of therapy is limited.

The functions of the testis are spermatogenesis, which takes place in the germinal epi-

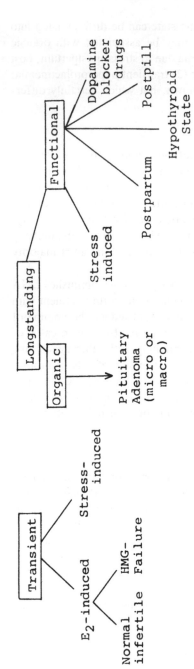

FIGURE 6.   Different types of hyperprolactinemia.

thelium of seminiferous tubules and steroidogenesis, which takes place in the interstitial cells (Leydig). The regulation of testicular function is controlled by an interaction between the CNS, hypothalamus, hypophysis, and testis. The spermatogenesis in man requires a period of 70 ± 5 d. The passage of sperm through the epididymis and vas deferens varies with the mean time of 12 d. It is not a single process of transport, but it is vital to allow further sperm maturation and development of sperm motility. The process of ejaculation is controlled by the nervous system and involves the secretion of prostate, testicular, and seminal vesicular components.

Disorders of male infertility may be classified as follows: (1) defect in sperm production, (2) defect in seminal plasma production, and (3) defect in sperm transport.

The etiological factors of testicular dysfunction associated with azoospermia (20% of infertile males) may be divided into the following categories:

1. Environmental factors due to exposure to noxious substances such as pharmacological agents, chemical preparations, cytotoxic drugs, insecticides, radiation, and emotional stress
2. Systemic diseases, endocrinopathies, infections, and vascular disorders
3. Genetic and developmental disorders
4. Iatrogenic factors such as heat, and following surgery, chemotherapy and androgenic therapy.

From 2 to 5% of all infertile men have a chromosomal abnormality. The most common cytogenetic disease is the Kleinfelter syndrome. Failure of onset of spermatogenesis, due to a primary germ aplasia (Sertoli cell only), is a relatively common condition. A male born with a bi- or unilateral undescended testis may have a defective spermatogenesis naturally in the undescended testis but also in the descended one.

Mumps orchitis at puberty may be responsible for 30% of males with disturbances in the spermatogenetic process. Azoospermia may be found in males who have undergone operative correction of bladder neck with uretheral reimplantation during childhood and in patients who were treated by chemotherapy and radiation for malignant diseases. Cases of testicular failure secondary to endocrinopathies like hypopituitarism due to a tumor or focal infection are of primary important to be diagnosed since they can benefit from the application of hormonal therapy. Defective sperm transport may be due to some mechanical block anywhere from the rete testis to the ejaculatory duct. The obstruction of the male reproductive tract may be caused by congenital malformation, postinfection (gonorrhea, tuberculosis), or surgery. Infection of seminal vesicles and the prostate may alter the quality, volume, and pH of the seminal fluid, which serves as a vehicle and provides protective and nutritive elements for spermatozoa. Varicocele of the spermatic veins, usually unilateral, is associated with decreased sperm count and lower sperm motility. Testicular biopsy from infertile patients with varicocele shows bilateral abnormalities characterized by hypoplasia of germinal cells and the presence of immature forms in the lumen of the seminiferous tubules.

The mechanism of normal ejaculation depends on the intact autonomic nervous system, and either chemical (α-adrenergic blocking preparations) or surgical sympathectomy can interfere with normal ejaculation. Sympathetic disturbances of ejaculation may cause a bladder neck dysfunction, which leads to retrograde emission of semen into the urinary bladder. Sexual dysfunction, the disability to achieve or maintain an erection, premature ejaculation, or difficulty in ejaculation may be etiological factors in infertility.

Medical history, clinical examinations, and sperm analysis should be the primary step in infertility evaluation (Figures 7 and 9). The semen analysis may be considered the most important test in the evaluation of male infertility, even though it is difficult to define a normal fertile ejaculate. There is no sharp line between fertility and infertility insofar as the parameters of semen quality are concerned.

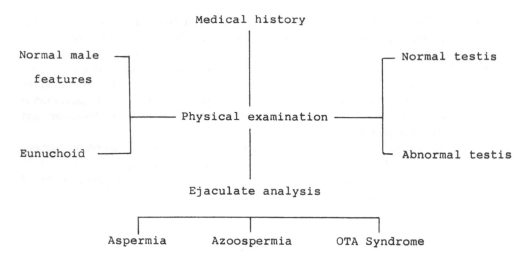

FIGURE 7.   Algorithmic approach to the evaluation of the male factor in infertility.

The examination of ejaculate is undertaken with regard to morphological, biochemical, and vitality aspects (Figure 8). Approximately 20% of infertile males are azoospermic. Azoospermia may be due to spermatogenic failure, obstruction of any level of the genital tract, or retrograde ejaculation. The algorithmic approach to the evaluation and treatment of the azoospermic male is shown in Figure 10. In most azoospermic males, there is little hope of restoring normal spermatogenesis. Only in cases of hypogonadotrophic hypogonadism was fertility achieved following administration of HMG-HCG therapy and more recently following application of Gn-RH analogs. Cryptorchidism is a potentially preventable cause of infertility, if the testis is brought into the scrotum early in life. When the epididimis or vas has become obstructed because of veneral disease, tuberculosis, or after acute nonspecific epididimitis, the obstruction can often by surgically corrected in about 40 to 50% of the cases. Pregnancies in cases of retrograde ejaculation were obtained following pharmacological therapy or recovery of sperm from the urinary bladder.

Semen with low concentration (oligospermia), impaired motility (asthenospermia), and morphologically abnormal (teratospermia) may be defined as the OTA syndrome (Figure 11). This is the most common form of male infertility disorder. Each of the factors of spermatozoa density, motility, and morphological abnormality can impair the process of procreativity. The degree of severity of each parameter can significantly differ in various patients. Among the factors that can play a major role in the development of this syndrome are primary testicular hypoplasia as in the undescended testis, atrophy of the testis due to trauma, inflammation, radiation, drugs, nicotine, chemical agents, heat, and varicocele. The main problem in the therapy of this condition is that the cause of reduced fertility is unknown and consequently, no specific therapy is available. Several hormones and drugs have been used with varied degrees of success. The different treatment approaches of empiric forms of therapy are hormonal preparations, HMG-HCG, CC, taxomophen, Gn-RH analogs, androgens, anti-inflammatory therapy with antibiotics and antiphlogistic preparation, immunosuppressive therapy with corticosteroids, use of andrenergic drugs, vitamins, caffeine, aspirin, zinc, kallikrein, etc. Recently, intrauterine insemination of sperm following washing and the use of different preparation procedures have been applied. In the presence of varicocele, surgical treatment of high ligation of spermatic vein has been applied. Semen quality improves in 50 to 60% of men following surgical procedure, but conception is achieved in only 35 to 30% of the cases. Recently, pregnancies were achieved by applying the new technology of IVF and GIFT procedure in cases with a low quality of semen. Sperm motility

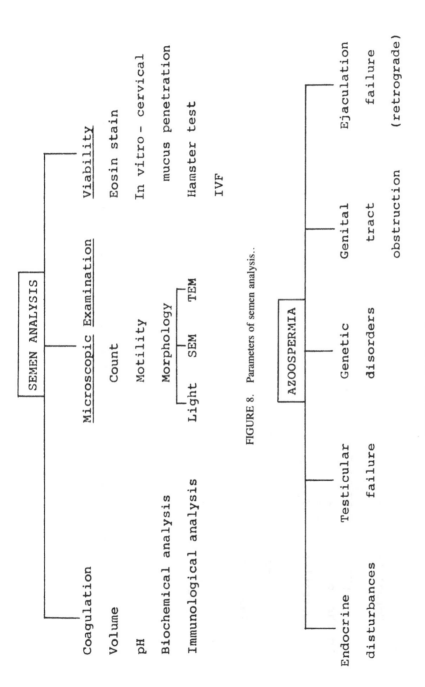

FIGURE 8. Parameters of semen analysis.

FIGURE 9. Etiology of azoospermia.

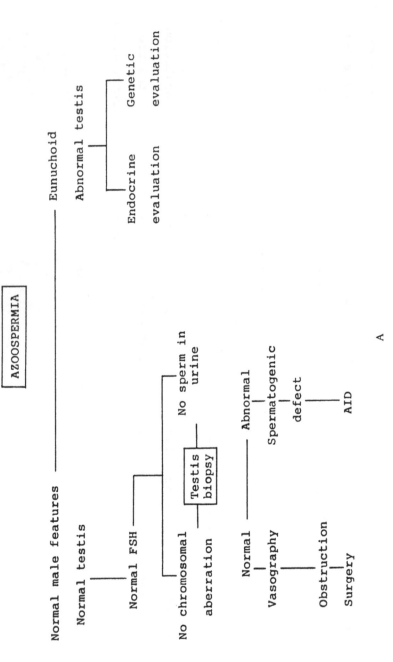

FIGURE 10. (A) Assessment and treatment of azoospermia. (B) Assessment and treatment of azoospermia.

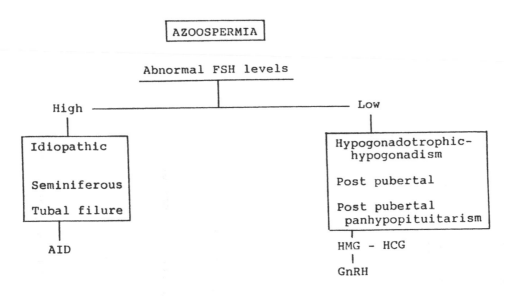

FIGURE 10B.

was the single most important parameter determining fertilization rate. Fertilization failed when motility of spermatozoa used was below 30%. The percentage of abnormal sperm forms had a negative effect on fertilization, but it was effective when there was more than 60% of abnormal forms. Sperm density had no effect on fertilization rate. In the future, clinical progress may be achieved by injecting one sperm into the perivitelline space or by drilling a hole in the zona pellucida by micromanipulation of the gametes.

Aspermia may be due to endocrine causes, retrograde ejaculation, and impotence (Figure 12).

VII. MECHANICAL FACTORS OF INFERTILITY

The physiological process of gamete transport from ovulation to intrauterine implantation requires a precise and coordinate function of the fallopian tubes and the ovaries. The mechanism involved in this function includes

1. Oocyte release from the ovary
2. Oocyte pick-up by the fimbriated end of the tube
3. Transport of the oocyte and sperm into the place of fertilization
4. Maintenance of the gametes and embryo in the tube during transport, fertilization, and cleavage
5. Transport of the embryo to the uterine cavity

It is obvious that a disruption in any of these functions could lead to infertility. This would be defined as mechanical infertility due to the inability of the potential conceptus to be formed and to reach the uterine cavity, given that there is a normal process of ovulation, either spontaneous or induced, normal sperm production, and no hostile cervical mucus or antisperm antibodies. The mechanical factor is second only to the male factor in contributing to infertility. It is involved in 30 to 35% of the cases.

The etiology of tubal malfunction can be due to many causes and varies widely in different countries. The most common cause is previous inflammatory disease leading to tubal obstruction and periadnexal adhesions. In our center, postinfection tubal damage is probably

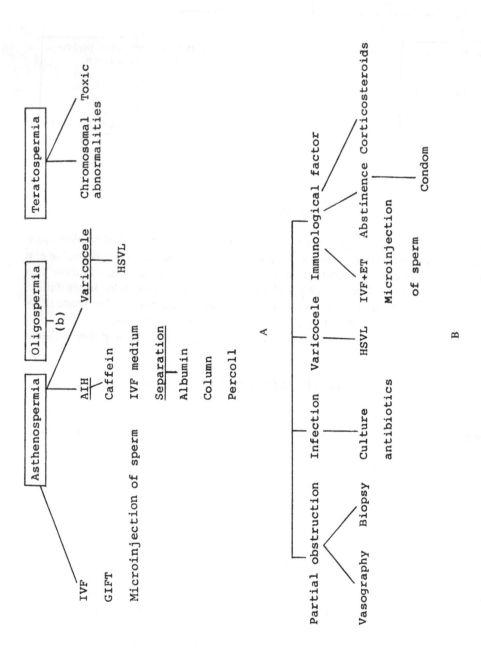

FIGURE 11.   (A) Etiology and therapeutic approach in cases of OTA syndrome. (B) Etiology and therapeutic approach in cases of oligospermia.

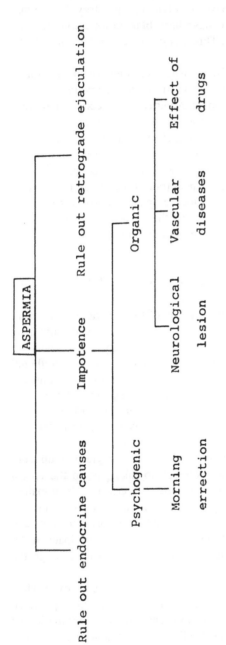

FIGURE 12. Etiological factors of aspermia.

the major cause of mechanical infertility, including previous interruption of pregnancy (23%), pelvic inflammatory disease unspecific (17.5%), and appendicitis (3.7%). Other causes were previous ovarian surgery (14%), endometriosis (5%), and previous tubal ligation (2.5%). The inflammatory process may be specific or nonspecific. The nonspecific infection, resulting from the spread of the microorganism from the vagina and the endocervix, is due to post-abortion, postpuerperal infection, a recently more common pelvic inflammatory disease that is associated with the use of IUD. Induced abortions have been blamed for a long time as being a predisposing factor for mechanical infertility. This was supported by several authors, but was not proved by others.

Salpingitis caused by microbacterium tuberculosis, parasites, or fungi is uncommon in developed countries. The incidence of genital tuberculosis is still high in some regions over the world like the Middle East, Africa, and part of South America. Gonoccocus and chlamydia are among the causative organisms transmitted by sexual activity causing mechanical infertility. Noninfectious causes of infertility include endometriosis, adhesions postpelvic surgery, congenital anomalies of the tubes, polyps, and calcified ectopic pregnancy.

Congenital abnormalities such as congenital absence of the tubes and reduplication are uncommon. Dysfunction of the tubes, which prevents gamete transport and that of the early conceptus, may be a cause of infertility even though the tubes are patent. Tubal dysfunction, which involves interference of peristalsis, cilial function, and the pick-up mechanism, may be caused by endocrine dysfunction, but is usually due to peritubal adhesions.

A. Pathophysiology of Mechanical Infertility

Postinfectious mechanical infertility can involve the tubal proximal and distal ends, the endosalpingeal mucosa, and peritubal and periovarian surfaces.

The impairment of fertility could arise from the malfunction of these various anatomical sites. Damage to the endosalpingeal mucosa can be responsible for deficient endosalpingeal secretions thus depriving the sperm, oocyte, and embryo of the necessary environment for survival. The ciliated cells at the fimbrial end represent more than 60% of the epithelial cells in the tubal mucosa, and in the ampulla, 40 to 60% of the cells are ciliated. Damage to the ciliary function could prevent the proper transport of the gametes and embryo along the tube. Intraluminal adhesions, although enabling passage of the sperm toward the oocyte, could prevent the transport of the growing embryo toward the uterus and result in the loss of the embryo or in tubal pregnancy.

Damage to the muscular layers of the tube impairs the tubal role in oocyte pick-up from the ovary, the tubal contraction movements that are believed to take part in the sperm migration into the tube and oocyte, and embryo transport toward the uterus may be impaired and the healing process that takes place ends eventually in tubal proximal or distal occlusion.

The formation of peritubal adhesions, together with its potential barrier formation between the tube and the ovary which interferes with oocyte pick-up, may also participate in the reduction of the functional motility of the tube and affect transport of gametes through the oviduct.

In pelvic endometriosis, the mucosal anatomy of the tubes is usually spared even when there are severe peritubal adhesions and agglutination of the fimbria. In hydrosalpinx, on the other hand, there is usually extensive damage to mucosal anatomy with diminution of the mucosal folds, significantly lower amounts of ciliated cells, and often abnormal secretory cells. Preservation of ciliary cells is of major importance for tubal function.

B. Assessment of Mechanical Infertility

1. Tubal Insuflation (Rubin Test)

The test entails the passage of CO_2 gas under pressure through the cervix to establish the patency of the genital tract. It is a simple ambulatory procedure which gives a fairly definitive indication of at least one tube patency or bilateral occlusion, organic or functional. Since it will not tell the type and localization of an obstruction, this test is not practiced at present. The procedure is not entirely without risk, and may cause pelvic inflammatory disease and complications resulting from inducing CO_2 under excessive pressure.

2. *Hysterosalpingography*

The value of hysterosalpingography (HSG) in fertility investigation is mainly the evidence it gives of the status of the cervical canal, the uterine cavity, and the tubal lumen. In the cervical canal, an occasional stenosis is discovered and dilated, or adhesions are diagnosed and later removed. The uterine cavity is delineated, possibly diagnosing intrauterine adhesions, polyps, submucus myomas, or tuberculosis showing an obliterated uterine cavity with vascular or myometrial intravasation of the contrast material, tubal obstruction, and tubal or ovarian calcifications. Tubal endometriosis showing a peculiar honeycomb pattern is an exclusive HSG finding. HSG also can detect tubal polyps and salpingitis isthmica nodosa. With the use of water-soluble contrast material, it is sometimes possible to evaluate the ampullary rugal pattern and the persistence of luminal folds indication (minimal or no endosalpingeal damage). It is a valuable assessment when reconstructive tubal surgery is considered. When proximal tubal obstruction is the case, HSG may help differentiate between organic obstruction and function spasm because in organic obstruction there often is extravasation and pointed contrast material at the uterine horns, while in functional spasms round horns are often documented. Functional spasms can be caused by irritant solutions, stress, or stimulation of the andrenergic nerves in the circular muscle layer at the uterotubal junction. Spasm can also occur because of the difference of temperature between the contrast material and the tissue or too rapid injection of the contrast material. In addition, variability in the internal diameter may allow filling of one tube before the other and thus give the false impression of unilateral occlusion.

HSG is contraindicated in the presence of active pelvic infection. Reactivation of pelvic infection may occur after the use of either oily or water-soluble media, but it should not necessarily be attributed to the media itself but rather the procedure.

Allergic reaction may occur especially when water-soluble media are used. Intravasation of oily media can be a serious complication. It can be avoided with some exception, by injection of the medium into the uterus in small amounts and under low pressure.

It is possible to reach the diagnosis regarding mechanical infertility with HSG, but the conclusive diagnosis of tuboperitoneal pathology should always be complimented by subsequent laparoscopic findings.

3. *Laparoscopy*

The first laparoscopic examination was performed by Jacobaus in 1910. In 1947, Palmer popularized laparoscopy for diagnostic procedures and from then it spread rapidly over the Western Hemisphere. The indication for laparoscopy is the evaluation of infertility in general, and especially the evaluation of tuboperitoneal pathology before performing reconstructive surgical procedures. Indications for surgical laparoscopy in infertility cases are lysis of adhesions, cauterization of endometriotic lesions, and occasional reconstructive tubal surgery.

Laparoscopy is usually performed under general anesthesia with endotracheal intubation, although local or epidural anesthesia can be applied. A small subumbilical incision is performed and a veres needle is inserted into the abdominal cavity at 40° toward the pelvis. Pneumoperitoneum is achieved by introduction of CO_2 with an insufflator that allows continuous monitoring of the flow pressure. After a satisfactory pneumoperitoneum is achieved with the optimal intra-abdominal pressure of 12 to 14 mmHg, the trocar is inserted at 45° angle toward the pelvis. As the insertion is a blind procedure technique, for open laparoscopy, especially in cases when intra-abdominal adhesions are suspected, optic pieces are used by some surgeons. With its fiber optic cable connected to a light source, the optic piece is inserted into the trocar sleeve and the pelvic cavity is inspected. Tubal patency is evaluated by installation of dye through a cervical cannula into the uterus and tubes. It is possible to introduce a second and sometimes a third instrument to assist the diagnostic procedure, and when surgical interventions such as adhesiolysis, tubal surgery, ovarian surgery, and surgical treatment of endometriosis are needed.

Most of the complications of laparoscopy occur during the phase of creation of pneumoperitoneum, sometimes related to anesthesia. Absolute contraindication to labaroscopy is a cardiopulmonary dysfunction of the patient. Other complications are CO_2 embolism, perforation and laceration of the bowel, injury to large blood vessels, and hemorrhage.

4. Hysteroscopy

Hysteroscopy has no practical use in the evaluation of tubal patency. It is an examination complementary to HSG and uterine curettage, providing direct visualization of the endocervical canal and the endometrial cavity. Hysteroscopy is indicated for diagnosis and localization of submucus fibroids, polyps, intrauterine adhesions, and abnormal uterine bleeding. It is most effective in the surgical treatment of septate uterus, pedunculated submucus myoma, lysis of intrauterine adhesions, and removal of a lost IUD or fragments of IUD.

Hysterscopy should not be performed in the presence of active pelvic inflammatory disease, during menstrual bleeding, and when intercourse took place between the last menstruation and the time of examination.

Some of the complications of the procedure are pelvic inflammatory disease, hemorrhage, and perforation of the uterus. When CO_2 is used, there is the risk of gas embolism, cardiac arrhythmias and arrest, and respiratory arrest, although these are very rare. With the use of Hyskon, there is the risk of an allergic reaction and circulatory overload.

Comparative studies between HSG and laparoscopy and between HSG and hysteroscopy established the value of each of these procedures in infertility investigation. HSG carries 25% incorrect diagnosis when it appears normal when a mechanical problem exists or by showing obstruction when the tubes are patent. Nevertheless, one cannot disregard the valuable information given by HSG concerning the uterine cavity, although it is not always as accurate as hysteroscopy, which confirms only 69% of abnormalities detected by HSG. In addition, the information regarding the lumen of the tubes is almost exclusive to HSG. In evaluation of the tuboperitoneal factor of infertility, laparoscopy is most effective when combined with HSG.

C. Surgical Treatment of Mechanical Infertility

Corrective surgical procedures were employed by infertility surgeons for many years. The aim of corrective surgery in mechanical infertility is the restoration of the anatomical and functional capacity of the reproductive organs to participate in the process of conception. For that purpose, various procedures are used, including resection of adhesions surrounding the tubes, ovaries, uterus, and bowel, salpingostomy for the restoration of tubal patency in cases of distal occlusion of the tubes, and tubal implantation or tubal anastomosis in cases with a proximal occlusion. In the past, most of the corrective infertility surgery was performed with conventional surgical methods. In the last 10 years, there has been a change in attitude with the introduction of microsurgical techniques that led to the concept that conventional surgery for delicate organs such as the fallopian tubes is a traumatic procedure. It results in tissue damage due to the cumbersome crushing instruments and rough suture material used. Tissue irrigation was used infrequently and the lack of magnification allowed only imprecise manipulations. In comparison, microsurgery employs fine instrument, very fine sutures, intense light and magnification, very gentle tissue handling, careful dissection and anastomosis, and accurate approximation of tissues, thus significantly reducing trauma to the tissue. A wide range of pregnancy rates following corrective infertility surgery was reported. After resection of adhesions by conventional surgery, the pregnancy rate reported was 20 to 57%, very similar to the 25 to 57% pregnancy rate reported by the microsurgeons. Also for salpingostomy, a wide range of success rates (14 to 41%) was reported by the conventional surgeons compared to 10 to 49% by the microsurgeons. For proximal tubal occlusion, tubocorneal implantation was usually used by the conventional surgeons with a success rate of 11 to 34%. The microsurgical approach to proximal occlusion is tubocorneal anastomosis with a pregnancy rate of 53 to 68%, and when tubotubal anastomosis was performed, a success rate of 37 to 80% was achieved.

The pregnancy rate following surgical treatment in cases of postinfectious tubal disease seems to be lower than the average microsurgical results, being only 18% after salpingostomy and 33% after anastomosis.

Comparing the results of conventional surgery to microsurgery, one may observe that the microsurgical approach is of significant value in some procedures, such as tubal anastomosis and tubocorneal anastomosis, but of limited value in resection of adhesions and salpingostomy.

Compared to the disappointing results of first tuboplasty, the results of repeated tuboplasty are even worse, with a 12 to 13% pregnancy rate.

Recently, some centers acquired experience with the use of a laser beam for microsurgery. This method offers the operator a well-controlled incision instrument with high maneuverability and precision and a bloodless operating field as the beam seals the blood vessels along its tract. The latter effect, on the other hand, also may be considered a disadvantage because of the thermal damage to the adjacent tissue. For this reason, some operators suggest the use of a laser for salpingostomy, adhesiolysis, and endometriosis, but not for tubal anastomosis.

D. Factors Affecting Prognosis

Experimental studies have shown that damage to the tubes, as caused by the inflammatory process reducing the ciliary and secretory activity in the tubes, is of major importance in the failure of surgical correction of the mechanical factor. Some authors have suggested taking biopsies from the endosalpinx for histological evaluation of the extent of damage, but biopsies are of limited prognostic value because of the different degrees of damage in various parts of the tube.

Inspection of the ampullary lumen under an operating microscope with the highest magnification was suggested for quantitative evaluation of the ciliary population and the tubal wall thickness. Mild tubal damage is diagnosed only if the thickness of the tubal wall is less than 1 mm and the ciliary cells account for at least 75% of the cell population. A wall thickness of 1 to 2 mm and cilia on 50 to 75% of the surface are indications of moderate damage, while the damage is severe if the wall thickness is more than 2 mm with severely reduced ciliary mucosa. Even dilated thin-walled hydrosalpings have a better prognosis than narrow lumen, thick-walled tubes. Therefore, the main factors affecting prognosis are the extent of tubal wall fibrosis and the extent of deciliation of the epithelial cell lining.

Various methods are used for the prevention of adhesion formation after surgery. Barrier substances like 10% of 32% dextran are left in the pelvis at the end of surgery. Medical treatment with dexamethasone and progesterone instilled in the pelvis at the end of surgery and administered parenterally during the postoperative period. Early postoperative laparoscopy for the dissection of newly formed adhesions is practiced by some surgeons.

E. Contraindications for Tubal Surgery

Contraindications for tubal surgery include genital tuberculosis, distal occlusion of the tubes with salpingitis isthmica nodosa, tubes less than 4 cm long or without fimbriae following previous surgery, active pelvic infection, nodular hydrosalpinx, persistence of intrauterine adhesions, diseases incompatible with pregnancy, ovulation failure refractory to ovulation induction, and age over 40 years.

Many attempts were made to classify the extent of tubal damage in order to choose the correct approach to mechanical infertility. The advent of an alternative such as IVF gave this issue a high priority as one should consider the chance of the patient to conceive after surgery with the alternative of IVF in mind.

F. *In Vitro* Fertilization

IVF of human oocytes and the establishment of pregnancies opened a new era in reproductive medicine with major improvements in the techniques of ovulation induction, monitoring of ovarian response, laboratory techniques of insemination, incubation, and embryo freezing. Although regarded initially only as the last chance for patients with uncorrectable tubal infertility, the indications for IVF treatment have expanded enormously to include male subfertility, immunological infertility, endometriosis, genital tuberculosis, unexplained infertility, and the problem of absent or nonfunctional ovaries that can now be solved by the use of donated oocytes.

Prerequisites for treatment are the patient having no contraindication for pregnancy, the presence of a uterus hospitable to pregnancy, ovaries with either spontaneous or inducible ovulation, and fertile sperm. The patient's age is also important, and an age over 40 to 42 years is in most centers a criterion for exclusion from IVF treatment as a result of poor success rate in IVF. Regular menstrual pattern is not a prerequisite, since the regularity of menstruation and the presence or absence of spontaneous ovulation did not affect IVF results. The majority of IVF patients have a mechanical factor of infertility due to various causes: (1) absent tubes due to successive ectopic pregnancies or removal of one or both tubes during surgery for ovarian cyst or surgical treatment of pelvic inflammatory disease; (2) severe damage to the fallopian tubes in which surgery has poor prognosis; and (3) history of failed tubal corrective surgery or patent tubes after such an operation but no conception.

Although the first IVF pregnancies were achieved in spontaneous cycles, there is a general agreement today that better results can be achieved with the induction of superovulation. Various protocols are used for the induction of ovulation for IVF. Initially, CC was used, but the addition of HMG to the CC protocol greatly improved the yield of the IVF programs. However, because of the antiestrogenic effects of CC and its potential inhibitory effect on the fertilization of oocytes, many prefer the use of HMG alone or purified FSH alone or the combination of FSH and HMG.

Ovarian response is monitored by daily measurements of serum estradiol levels and ultrasonographic measurements of follicular growth. Many programs also monitor LH and progesterone levels to detect an early luteinization and premature ovulation. HCG is usually administered for the final maturation of oocytes when the ovarian response meets the prerequisite parameters of oocyte maturation. Oocyte pick-up is performed 36 h after HCG administration or 24 to 28 h after a spontaneous LH surge.

G. Oocyte Pick-Up Techniques

Laparoscopic oocyte pick-up (OPU) with follicular aspiration under vision and ultrasonically guided OPU are the current methods for OPU.

Laparoscopy was originally used and is still used by many centers for OPU, employing the three-puncture technique after induction of pneumoperitoneum and general anesthesia. However, lately the ultrasonically guided oocyte collection has become the method of choice in many centers. Comparative studies have shown the ultrasound technique to be as effective as laparoscopy in the number and quality of the oocytes recovered and the pregnancy rates.

Various approaches are used with this method, including the transabdominal-transvesical, the perurethral, and the transvaginal approaches. All these methods are similarly effective and well accepted by the patients, especially because local anesthesia can be employed for these procedures.

The ultrasound procedure is safe, easy to perform, and can be used as an outpatient procedure.

The oocytes recovered are inseminated according to maturity after a period of incubation which extends from 2 to 8 h for the mature oocytes to 24 h for the immature oocytes. Embryos are transferred to the uterus in a teflon catheter 40 to 44 h after insemination at a 2- to 8-cell stage. Usually three to four embryos are transferred and the spare embryos are frozen for a later transfer.

H. Selection of the Appropriate Treatment for Mechanical Infertility

The majority of patients referred to as IVF patients had tubal corrective surgery in the past which failed to restore patency. In some cases, surgery succeeded, but the patient did not conceive. It is obvious, in view of the low pregnancy rates of the repeated tubal surgery, that IVF offers these patients a better chance to achieve pregnancy; the current pregnancy rate in IVF is 20 to 30%. Patients who need only adhesiolysis or reanastomosis post-tubal ligation, where the pregnancy rates reach up to 57 to 80%, clearly benefit more from microsurgery. For the remainder of the patients with mechanical infertility who need salpingostomy, anastomosis, or tubal implantation, the odds of success in achieving pregnancy with microsurgery are probably not superior today to those with IVF, and it should be left to clinical judgment whether to refer them to microsurgery or IVF.

Selection of patients for tubal surgery or IVF may improve pregnancy rates for the surgical procedure and avoid surgery in cases with poor prognosis where IVF obviously offers a better chance. A balance should be established between surgery and IVF since surgery, when successful, has a major advantage in enabling the patient to conceive more than once after a single operation, while with the 20 to 30% pregnancy rate offered today by the IVF procedure, the patient may have to be submitted for the procedure a number of times before pregnancy is likely to occur. Surgery also offers better pregnancy rates in mild cases. On the other hand, there are many advantages of IVF over tubal surgery. Among these are a lower operative risk, a short hospital stay, and low cost (Figure 13).

VIII. IMMUNOLOGICAL CAUSES OF INFERTILITY

Immunological causes of infertility have been recognized for a long time. However, a systemic approach with a universally standardized laboratory work-up is still lacking. Sperm antibodies play a major role in immunollogical infertility. Human seminal plasma is reached in antigens. The spermatozoa itself possesses antigens on the acrosom, midpiece and tail, which may contribute to immunological infertility. Sperm enzymes contribute to antigenicity of the sperm. Those antigens may provoke local and/or systemic antibody response. In the female reproductive tract, antibodies may be detected in the cervical, endometrial, and tubal environment. This may be secreted locally or arise as a transudate from plasma. Antibodies may interfere with sperm motility, cause agglutination, reduce adherence to zona, and subsequently interfere with fertilization. Autoantibodies in the male likewise may be found either in the seminal plasma, the systhemic circulation, or both. Theoretically, immune response may impede implantation and fetal development. The most important aspect of sperm-related antibodies is that they may reduce, but not necessarily abolish, fertility. Proper interpretation of laboratory tests and clinical results is impossible without recognizing the fact that some of the antibody tests are not specific, especially those that rely upon agglutination reaction. Various treatment schedules were attempted in the treatment of immu-

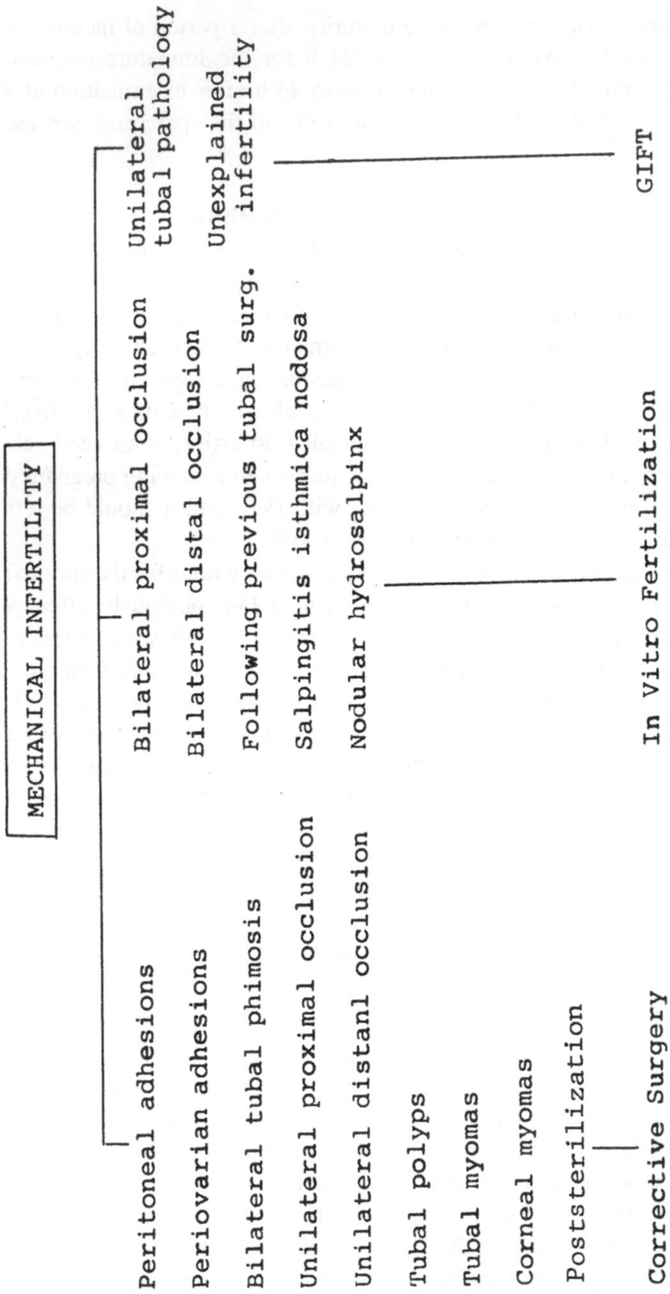

MECHANICAL INFERTILITY

Peritoneal adhesions
Periovarian adhesions   Bilateral proximal occlusion   Unilateral
Bilateral tubal phimosis   Bilateral distal occlusion   tubal pathology
Unilateral proximal occlusion Following previous tubal surg. Unexplained
Unilateral distanl occlusion   Salpingitis isthmica nodosa   infertility
Tubal polyps   Nodular hydrosalpinx
Tubal myomas
Corneal myomas
Poststerilization

Corrective Surgery   In Vitro Fertilization   GIFT

FIGURE 13.   Selection of first choice therapeutic approach in mechanical infertility.

nological infertility (Figure 14). Immunosuppressive therapy with high doses of corticosteroids to either of both partners and prolonged use of condoms resulted in occasional success. Attempts to remove antisperm antibodies by sperm washing before intrauterine insemination may have some benefit; however, the high affinity of antisperm antibodies probably precludes effective sperm washing. Rapid dilution of the ejaculate is another *in vitro* sperm manipulation that may be of benefit. Recently, few encouraging reports demonstrated a successful treatment of immunological infertility by IVF and ET.

IX. UNEXPLAINED INFERTILITY

Unexplained infertility should be applied to couples who failed to achieve conception despite the most thorough evaluation that discovered no obvious cause for their infertility or after correction of any factor that may be responsible for infertility. In that sense, unexplained infertility may be diagnosed in a normal female whose husband is azoospermic and fails to conceive with donor insemination. The incidence of unexplained infertility varies between 6 to 27% and is universally related to the thoroughness of the infertility evaluation. In order to apply the term of unexplained infertility, one should reveal many subtle causes of infertility like sperm incorporation through ooplasma of zona-free Hamster eggs (SPA), transient hyperprolactinemia, luteal phase defects, androgen excess, and Luft syndrome. Occult infection in mycoplasma and chlamydia belong to the same category, and immunological factors should also be ruled out.

At present, in cases of unexplained infertility, IVF and ET or GIFT procedures should be applied.

X. PSYCHOLOGICAL CAUSE OF INFERTILITY

Infertility is at present not socially acceptable in societies of developed and developing countries. An infertile couple is under severe social pressure in most societies. Emotional factors as causes of infertility can be attributed to less than 5% of the couples.

Emotional stress, mediated by the hypothalamic-pituitary-gonadal axis, may result in ovulatory disorders such as amenorrhea and progesterone deficiency.

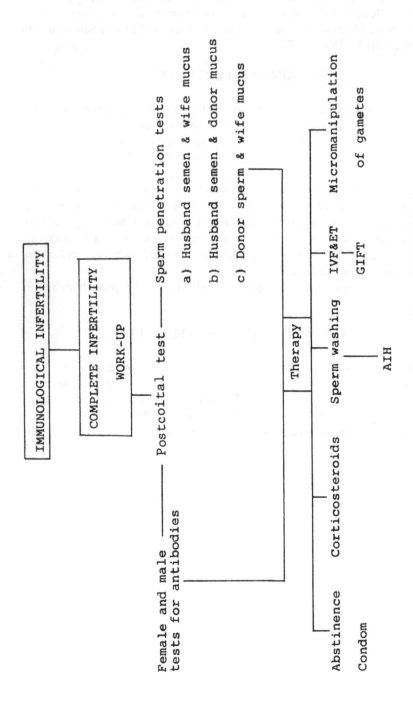

FIGURE 14.   Assessment and treatment of immunological infertility.

Chapter 3

NORMAL ANATOMY OF THE FEMALE PELVIS AND SONOGRAPHIC DEMONSTRATION OF PELVIC ABNORMALITIES

Davor Jurkovic and Asim Kurjak

TABLE OF CONTENTS

I. INTRODUCTION

An accurate knowledge of the sonographic anatomy of the female pelvis is a basic pre-requisite for detection of any abnormality. By distension of the urinary bladder, gas-filled bowel loops are displaced from the lesser pelvis permitting the visualization of the genital organs and the anatomical structures within the lesser pelvis.[1] If gas in the rectosigmoid colon disturbs visualization of the posterior aspect of the uterus, a water enema may be utilized to allow visualization of the whole lesser pelvis content.[2] However, there are still some patients in whom quality of the image remains unsatisfactory. In such cases, a diffuse accumulation of echoes with poor definition of deep structures can be attributed to the increased amount of mesenteric fat in the pelvis, and these patients should be offered alternative imaging procedures.[3]

By using static equipment it is possible to obtain a clear overview of the whole pelvic content, including the anterior skeletal surface and pelvic musculature.[4] This more clearly illustrates anatomical relationships, which are sometimes difficult to appreciate on the limited "keyhole" views obtained with real-time machines.

The most significant advantage of real time is the ease of maneuverability, whereby one can quickly change scan planes and rapidly survey the pelvis, getting a three-dimensional impression of the structure under investigation. Another advantage of real time is the visualization of vascular pulsations and peristalsis, which may be helpful for the detection of the ovaries and prevents the misinterpretation of a fluid-filled bowel loop as an ovarian mass. This can occur when static equipment is used alone.[5]

The examination technique is more or less the same, regardless of whether static or real-time equipment is used. With the patient lying supine, the probe is placed suprapublically, and parallel transverse and longitudinal scans are performed. Oblique scans are then employed for a better delineation of a particular structure. The number of scans is practically unrestricted and examination time is much shorter when a real-time machine is used. It should be noted that the smaller scanning heads of real-time mechanical sector scanners represent an improvement over the larger, rectangular linear array probes, allowing easier accessibility to the sidewalls of the pelvis. As far as the frequency of the transducer is concerned, it is well known that it is always the rule in ultrasound to use the highest frequency transducer compatible with adequate penetration of the part being examined.[6] Most adult female pelves, however, can be adequately scanned using a 3.5- or 5.0-MHz transducer with either a medium or long internal focus.

A. Urinary Bladder

The most prominent organ on an ultrasound scan is the anteriorly located urinary bladder, which appears as an anechoic structure with thin walls. Its shape depends above all on the quantity of urine in it, the section level, and the obesity of the patient. If the bladder is not sufficiently full, it may hang from one or both sides of the uterus and imitate ovarian cysts (Figures 1 and 2).

In 60% of the patients, it is possible to observe dynamic movements within the bladder during examination. This so-called "jet phenomenon" was explained by the different osmolality and specific gravity of the fresh urine injected from ureters and fluid within the bladder, and can be potentially useful in diagnosis of unilateral kidney disease (Figure 3).[7]

B. Uterus

The uterus is centrally located in the female pelvis, and is the most accessible organ for ultrasound evaluation. Uterine assessment includes its position, size, shape, contour, texture, and the appearance of the uterine cavity. Slight angulation of the uterine body to either the right or left is commonly seen in normal subjects. The corpus is usually anteflected to the

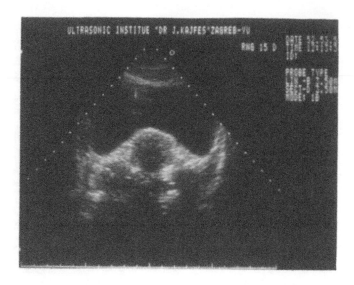

FIGURE 1. An example of an insufficiently full bladder that hangs from both sides of the uterus.

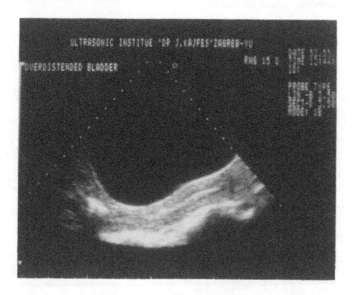

FIGURE 2. A case of an overdistended bladder. Note the elongated and thin appearance of the uterus.

cervix. In cases of retroflection, the uterus is more difficult to assess and can be easily misinterpreted as a pathological finding by an unexperienced operator (Figures 4 to 6).[8]

Uterine size and shape are mostly dependent on the patient's age and parity. Standards of uterine size have been described in numerous reports including the neonates, premenarcheal girls, and postpubertal and postmenopausal women.[9-12] In girls up to 7 years of age, the uterine size is not influenced by age and the cervix is relatively predominant over the corpus (Figure 7). Thereafter, the uterus increases steadily in size, and the corpus gradually becomes larger than the cervix, as in postpubertal women.[13] It is generally accepted that in normal nulligravidous women, the uterine size is up to 7 cm in longitudinal diameter and up to 4 cm in width and height. In multiparous women, all uterine diameters are on average 1.2 cm greater.[14] There are also slight variations in the uterine size during the cycle.[15]

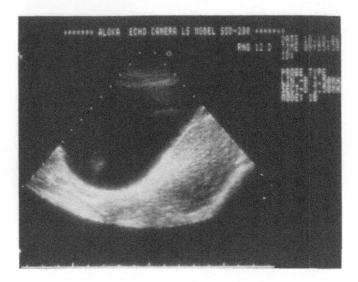

FIGURE 3.   Longitudinal scan of the uterus and vagina showing "jet phenomenon" within the bladder.

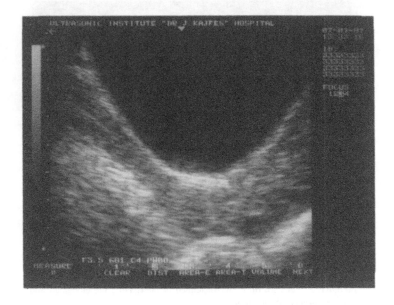

FIGURE 4.   Longitudinal scan of the vagina and uterine cervix. The mucosal attachment of the vagina produces a strong, thin linear echo.

The normal uterus has a well-defined contour and a pear-shaped configuration. The texture of the myometrium can be clearly demonstrated by current gray-scale equipment and is characterized by low to medium echogenicity.[16] The uterine shape, contour, and internal texture should be carefully evaluated in every patient because minor pathological changes can change some of the characteristics of a normal uterus before their clear visualization and distinction due to small size become possible.

Recently, the sonographic appearance of the endometrial cavity in particular has been studied. First reports described the endometrium as a prominent central cavity echo, which was the only endometrial feature visible by instruments of relatively poor resolution capa-

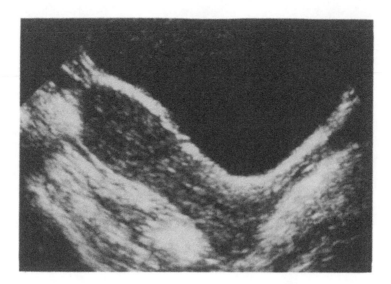

FIGURE 5.   Longitudinal scan of a normal uterus and vagina. The uterus is anteverted and the fundus is more anterior than the cervix. The uterine fundus is larger than the cervix.

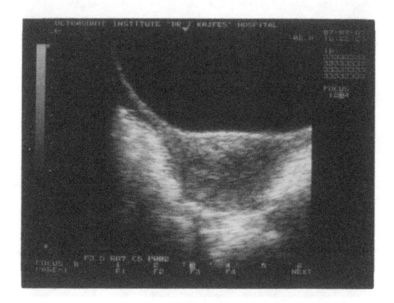

FIGURE 6.   Transverse sonogram of a normal uterus. The contour is clearly outlined and the texture displays homogeneous and moderate echogenicity.

bilities.[17,18] Further work has shown that phasic changes in the appearance of the endometrium can be recognized in 95 to 99% of patients, and typical findings in the proliferative and secretory phase have been described.[19-21] The characteristic appearance of the preovulatory endometrium is well known as the "ovulation ring" and serves as an additional parameter for better prognosis and detection of ovulation by ultrasound (Figures 8 to 10).[22]

C. Vagina

In contrast to the uterus, which is demonstrated in great detail on ultrasound examination, the vagina appears as a simple bright linear echo located below the bladder. This strong

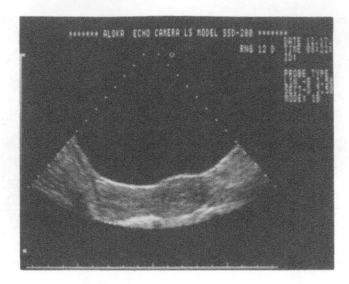

FIGURE 7.   Longitudinal scan of the prepubertal uterus. Note the predominance of the cervix over the corpus.

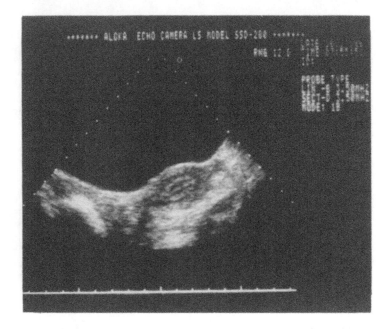

FIGURE 8.   Typical appearance of the preovulatory endometrium exhibiting increased basal layer echogenicity.

echo, measuring 7 to 10 cm in length, corresponds to the attached superficial layers of mucosa and is surrounded by the hypoechoic vaginal walls. If some fluid is present within the vagina, e.g., menstrual blood or urine, the linear echo is partially or completely absent, allowing its simple detection (Figure 11).

D. Adnexa

The adnexa consist of the broad ligament, fallopian tubes, mesosalpinx, and ovaries. The fallopian tubes and the broad ligament are rarely seen as a moderately hypoechoic area

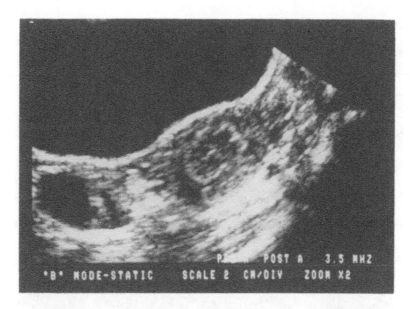

FIGURE 9. Another example of the preovulatory endometrium appearance.

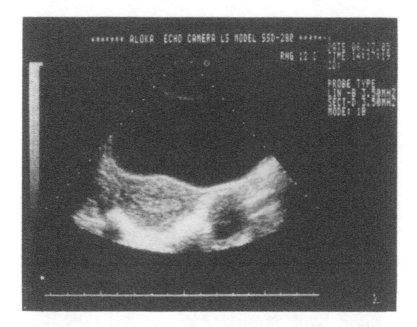

FIGURE 10. Echogenic endometrium in the secretory phase. The endometrium is thick and the central echo is lost.

extending laterally from the uterine fundus and measuring a few millimeters in thickness. Sometimes the adnexa may appear unusually prominent and more than 2 cm thick. It has been shown that this finding does not imply the presence of a pelvic inflammatory disease and has no clinical significance.[23] In more than 99% of cases, the ovaries are visible if current high-resolution real-time equipment is used.[24] The location of the ovaries is extremely variable in normal subjects because of their flexible attachment to the uterus and lateral pelvic wall. For this reason, it is quite unusual to demonstrate both ovaries in one transverse section. If the uterus is inclined to the right or left, one ovary is seen close to, or even

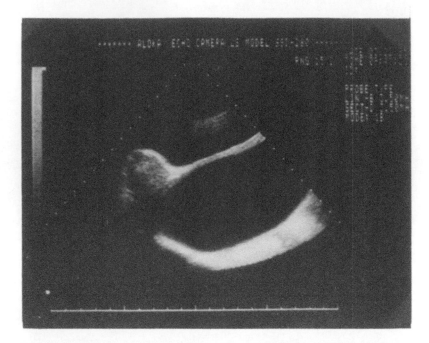

FIGURE 11.   Longitudinal sonogram of a patient with an imperforate hymen. The large cystic structure representing a hematocolpos and the small uterus are demonstrated.

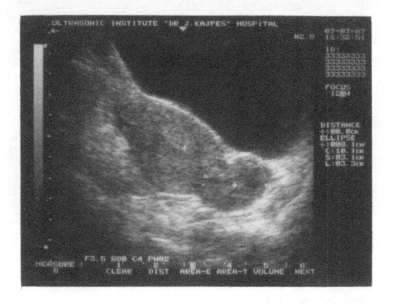

FIGURE 12.   The oblique scan through the left ovary exhibits normal shape and texture.

behind, the uterus, while the contralateral one is positioned laterally at variable distance. In retroflected uterus cases, the ovaries are typically located anteriorly and superiorly to the uterine fundus (Figure 12).[11] In such cases, pulsations in the internal iliac and ovarian arteries may be used as landmarks for assisting in ovarian identification.[25]

Normal ovaries are of fusiform shape and their size varies according to the age of the patient (Figures 13 and 14). In women of generative age, the usual size of the ovary is 3

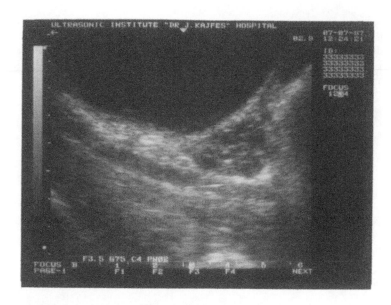

FIGURE 13. A case of a laterally positioned ovary. External iliac artery passing along the lateral pelvic wall is also demonstrated.

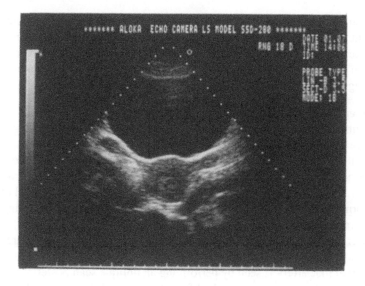

FIGURE 14. A case of uterine retroflection with the ovaries typically located above the uterine fundus.

cm in transverse length, 2 cm in anteroposterior length, and 1 cm in height. However, because of marked variability in ovarian shape and linear measurements, it would be more accurate to define ovarian volume according to the formula for a prolate elipse ($V = 0.5233 \times D_1 \times D_2 \times D_3$).[11] In premenarcheal girls, ovarian volume is relatively constant until 6 years of age, being below 1 ml. From that age, the ovarian volume rises and reaches a mean value of 4 ml at 13 years.[13] In the postpubertal group, the volume of the normal ovaries should be between 2 and 6 ml.[11] Postmenopausal ovaries, as has been shown in large series, are of similar size.[5] Ovarian size can also be estimated by calculating the ovarian surface or uterine-to-ovarian ratio.[26,27]

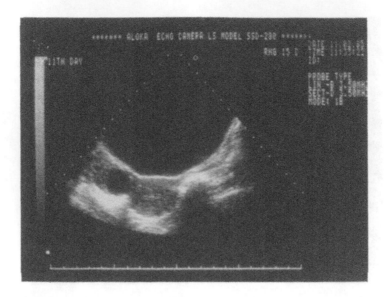

FIGURE 15.   Transverse sonogram of the uterus and the right ovary showing
a developing follicle. The follicle appears as a small and round cystic structure
with well-defined walls and clear fluid within.

The ovaries are generally hypoechoic compared to the uterus because of the multiple small follicles present in the cortical area. The medulla and capsule exhibit a higher echogenicity compared to the cortex. The growing follicle is easily demonstrated as a hypoechoic cystic structure within the ovarian substance, with a well-defined wall and a characteristic daily growth rate (Figure 15).

E. Other Lesser Pelvic Structures

Other anatomical structures that can be consistently demonstrated by sonography within lesser pelvis are the pelvic musculature and blood vessels. Visualization of these structures is less important from a clinical standpoint. The obturator internus muscle occupies a large part of the anterior and lateral pelvic walls and is demonstrated as a well-defined hypoechoic ovoid structure. The levator ani muscle is seen on a transverse scan at the level of the cervix and vaginal fornices and denotes the pelvic diaphragm. Other muscles forming the pelvic diaphragm are rarely seen because of their deep position.

Pelvic vessels are much more clearly defined on an ultrasound scan. They are sonographically demonstrated as tubular structures characterized by an anechoic lumen and hyperechoic walls. The internal iliac artery is seen by performing an oblique scan posteriorly and laterally to the ovaries. It can be easily distinguished from the internal iliac vein, which is typically located posterior to the artery. If a real-time machine is used, pulsations of the artery are easily seen while the diameter of the vein is constant. The external iliac artery and vein are also routinely imaged on an oblique scan directed through the bladder to the contralateral pelvic wall. The external iliac vein sometimes can be compressed by an overfull urinary bladder, so that only the artery is visualized. The ovarian artery approaches the ovary from its lateral and posterior aspect, and being relatively thin, is not regularly seen. However, meticulous scanning of the lateral periovarian space will demonstrate in 60 to 70% of examined women the ovarian artery and vein which reach the ovaries via the mesovarium. Because of their small diameter and variable ovarian position, it is difficult to distinguish between the artery and vein. Although there were several reports describing marked dilatation of the ovarian vessels at the periovulatory phase of the cycle,[25] we were not able to confirm this in spite of systematic scanning of patients during the late follicular phase of the cycle until ovulation (Figures 16 to 20).[28]

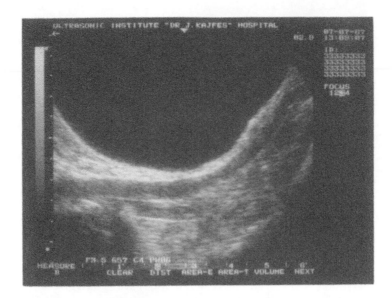

FIGURE 16.   External iliac artery as seen on an oblique scan directed to the lateral pelvic wall. The wall of the vessel is highly echogenic, while the lumen is anechoic.

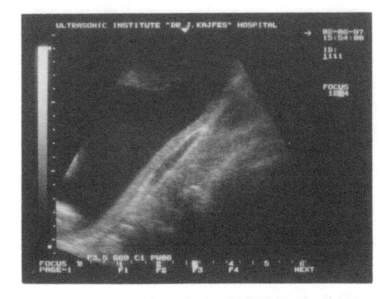

FIGURE 17.   Another example of ultrasound demonstration of the external iliac artery.

The ureters can also be routinely imaged in the lesser pelvis through a distended bladder.[29] The ureters are best seen by performing a longitudinal scan posterior to the ovaries, but may be also seen in transverse view. After entering the lesser pelvis, they are lying medial and anterior to the internal iliac vessels and continue caudally to insert into the trigone of the bladder. Any gross pelvic pathology of the uterus or ovaries may cause ureteral obstruction, so it is advisable to check its diameter during a routine examination.

II. SONOGRAPHIC DEMONSTRATION OF PELVIC ABNORMALITIES

Meticulous examination of the pelvis by ultrasound can very often show the underlying

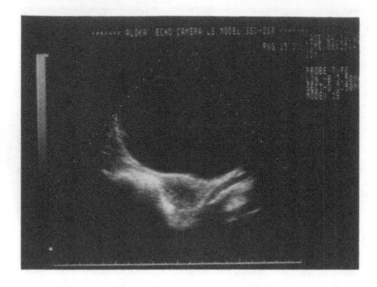

FIGURE 18.   Internal iliac artery on the left passing laterally to the uterus.

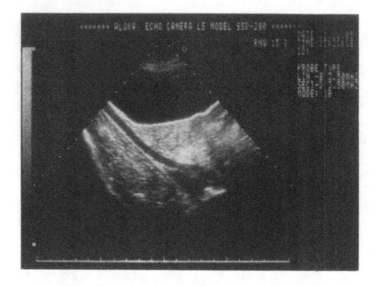

FIGURE 19.   Another example of clear visualization of the internal iliac artery.

cause of infertility. This chapter will, however, briefly describe present possibilities of ultrasound in diagnosing various pelvic pathologies, particularly those that can interfere with female fertility.

A. Uterine Abnormalities
1. Congenital Uterine Abnormalities
Congenital uterine abnormalities are strongly associated with infertility and habitual spontaneous abortion. The incidence of congenital uterine abnormalities has been estimated to be between 0.1 to 12%.[30,31] Since these conditions may cause serious complications in pregnancy (e.g., permature deliveries, abruptio placentae, or rupture of the uterus), their diagnosis in a nonpregnant subject is particularly valuable (Figures 21 to 23).

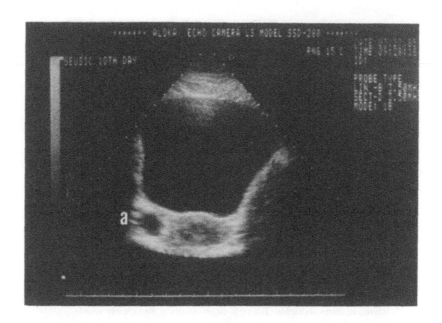

FIGURE 20. Ovarian artery (a) reaching the right ovary from the lateral side.

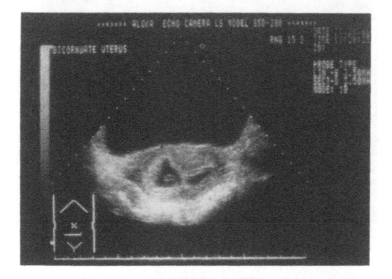

FIGURE 21. Transverse sonogram of a 7-week gestation showing the gestational sac in the right horn of a bicornuate uterus. The left horn is empty and clearly visible.

Until recently, hysterosalpingography was the only imaging technique for identifying uterine anomalies, however, now it cannot be accepted as a satisfactory screening method, particularly in the pediatric and adolescent female.[32] Congenital uterine anomalies are usually classified in three groups — agenesis, failure of cavitation, and failure of fusion being the most common. Accurate ultrasound diagnosis of fusion anomalies in a pregnant patient during the first trimester and the first half of the second trimester usually poses no difficulties, and has been reported extensively.[33,34] Ultrasonic diagnosis of these conditions in a non-

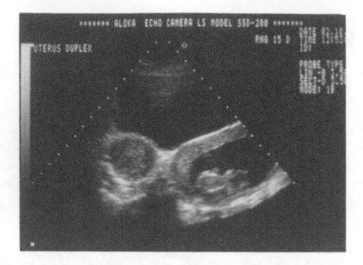

FIGURE 22. Transverse scan showing a 11-week-old pregnancy in the left uterus of uterus didelphis. The right empty uterus is also clearly visible.

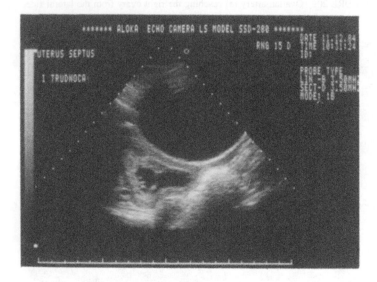

FIGURE 23. An 8-week pregnancy in a septate uterus. The gestational sac is situated in the right part of the uterine cavity and is separated by a thin membrane from the left part of the cavity, which is filled with blood.

pregnant patient seems to be less accurate when static equipment is used.[35] In our experience, if a high-resolution real-time mechanical sector is employed, one can attain such diagnostic accuracy that ultrasonography can be considered an ideal method for screening for uterine anomalies. As uterine anomalies regularly affect the ultrasonic appearance of the endometrial cavity, clear visualization of the endometrium is a guide to diagnosis. The examinations should be regularly performed in the secretory phase of the cycle when the endometrium is strongly echogenic and naturally contrasts with the hypoechoic myometrium. After accurate delineation of uterine position, scanning is performed in an entirely transverese uterine plane,

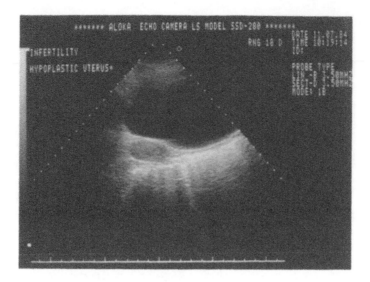

FIGURE 24. Hypoplastic uterus in a case of severe ovarian insufficiency. The endometrium is hardly recognizable.

starting from the level of the cervix and progressing superiorly by a slow, continuous movement. If there is a fusion anomaly present, one can clearly observe the splitting of the unique endometrial echo in the upper uterine portions.

This is characteristic for an arcuate, subseptate, and bicornuate uterus. Differential diagnosis to septate uterus or uterus didelphis usually poses no difficulties, because in these cases one can easily see two separate cervical canals or the splitting of the entire uterine cavity. More information about the type of abnormality is obtained by assessment of the myometrium. In bicornuate uterus and uterus didelphis it forms two separate horns, while in other anomalies it appears normal. However, any detected anomaly that has potential clinical significance should be confirmed by hysterosalpingography (Figures 24 to 27).

2. Uterine Fibroids (Leiomyomata)

The most common acquired anomaly of the uterus are uterine fibroids or leiomyomata, which are present in more than 20% of all women over 35 years of age.[36] The sonographic diagnosis of uterine fibroma is based on texture changes, distortion of the uterine contour, and uterine enlargement. The typical ultrasound image of fibroma is that of a hypoechoic intrauterine mass that affects the homogenicity of the normal uterine contour. Uterine enlargement is relatively constant, but not a pathognomonic sign of uterine fibroma. The uterus may be generally enlarged and present globular contours; conversely, separate nodules can be seen with a lobular uterine contour. It has been shown that uterine enlargement occurs in 66% of cases of histologically proven fibromas, while contour distortion and textural changes are seen in 76 and 68% of cases, respectively.[37] Contour distortion seems to be the most sensitive parameter of tumor presence, unless it is large enough to be visualized as a distinctive mass (Figure 28).

Nonetheless, the ultrasound diagnosis of fibroma is considered simple and accurate. The reported rate of specific histologic diagnosis by ultrasound was 65%.[38] The major cause of nonspecificity of sonographic findings is the presence of pedunculated tumors that are sometimes hardly distinguished from solid adnexal mass (Figures 29 to 31).

However, it should be remembered that leiomyomas are usually easily accessible for palpation, and the diagnosis of clinically significant tumors is in most cases made merely by palpation. Therefore, the need for ultrasound investigation of the fibroma can be easily

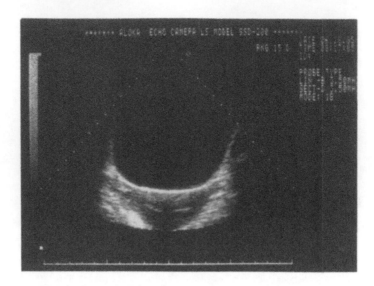

FIGURE 25.   Typical appearance of an arcuate uterus recognized as the division of the central cavity echo in the upper portions.

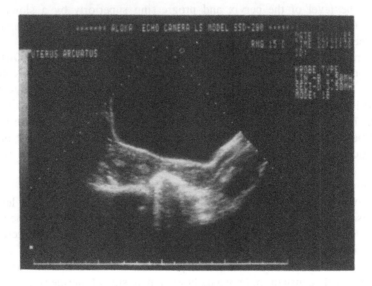

FIGURE 26.   Another example of an arcuate uterus.

reduced to cases in that either the palpatory findings are unclear or further information is required (e.g., in obese patients, difficult vaginal examination, a combination of fibroma with other tumors, follow-up of smaller tumors to evaluate more precisely their growth, and more accurate localization of myomatous knots).

Ultrasonic visualization of a uterine fibroid provides in a number of cases a fast and simple diagnosis of the cause of infertility. Infertility is the only symptom in a considerable amount of patients with a uterine fibroid. Large nodes in the posterior uterine wall dislocate the tubes and diminish their motility, so that acceptance and transport of fertilized ova are impossible. Nodes situated close to the sotia tubae uterine can cause mechanical obstruction of the tubes, and submucosal fibromas interfere with nidation.[39]

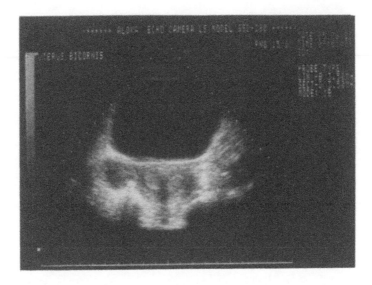

FIGURE 27. Uterus bicornis unicollis. The transverse section displays two distinct uterine cavities and two separate uterine horns.

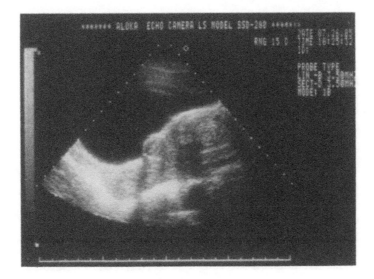

FIGURE 28. Longitudinal sonogram of the uterus with multiple small myomas. Note irregularity of the anterior uterine contour, which represents the most sensitive parameter for diagnosing tumor presence.

Differential diagnosis of uterine fibroma to sarcoma can be difficult. The common sonographic appearance of sarcoma is an enlarged uterus with an inhomogeneous texture. As secondary tumor changes often occur, large anechoic areas representing hemorrhage and necrosis are always seen.[40] Sonography is most helpful in the demonstration of the fast growth of previously detected fibroma, particularly in a postmenopausal patient (Figure 32).

B. Ovarian and Other Adnexal Masses

A common problem in clinical practice is sonographic diagnosis of adnexal mass. Accuracy of ultrasound in the evaluation of pelvic masses has been reported to be as high as 91 to

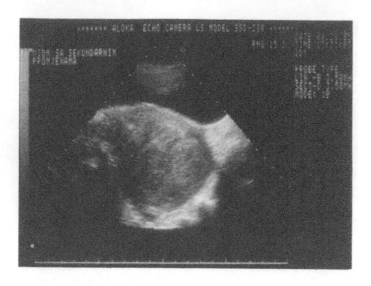

FIGURE 29.   Large uterine myoma with secondary changes: degeneration, calcification, and necrosis.

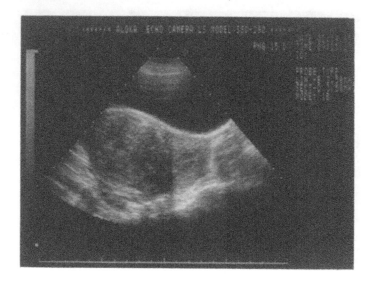

FIGURE 30.   Another example of a large uterine myoma with secondary changes.

97%.[40,41] When ultrasonic findings were compared with histomorphology after surgery, in the majority of cases, sonographic data about the presence, size, location, and internal consistency of the mass correlated well with pathological findings (Figures 33 and 34).[42]

Although there were several attempts to establish characteristic sonographic patterns of certain adnexal masses, particularly in cases of ovarian cystadenoma and dermoid cysts,[43,44] other authors described less encouraging experiences.[45,46] Therefore, it is generally accepted that ultrasonography does not reveal information about the histology of the tumor and, consequently, cannot provide a definitive clinical diagnosis.[47] Accordingly, the most rational approach presumes meticulous analysis of the morphological characteristics of the mass,

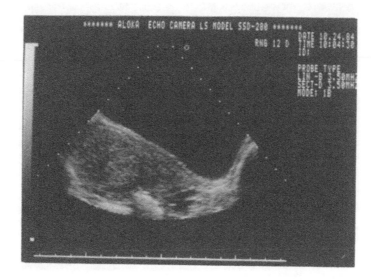

FIGURE 31.   Uterine sonogram demonstrating the uterine body on the left and a subserous myoma (on the right) appearing as a solid adnexal tumor.

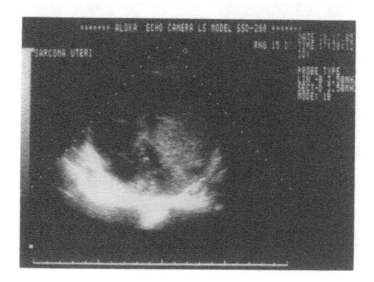

FIGURE 32.   Extremely large uterine tumor with pronounced degeneration, necrosis, and hemorrhage. The diagnosis of uterine sarcoma was confirmed on laparotomy.

including its origin, size, texture, and relationships to the other pelvic organs. Criteria for the sonographic assessment of adnexal masses have been developed by Fleischer et al.,[48] and if interpreted together with relevant clinical data, enable considerable reduction of diagnostic possibilities (Figures 35 to 38).

A particular problem in that field is the diagnosis of ovarian malignancy, which represents 25% of all gynecological malignancies. It has been reported that certain sonographic features like thick septa and solid nodules are highly suggestive of malginancy,[49] and the likelihood of malignancy increases proportionally to the amount of solid echogenic material within the

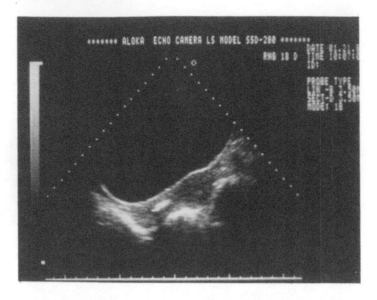

FIGURE 33.   Longitudinal scan showing highly echogenic sinechia in the cervical canal in an infertile patient.

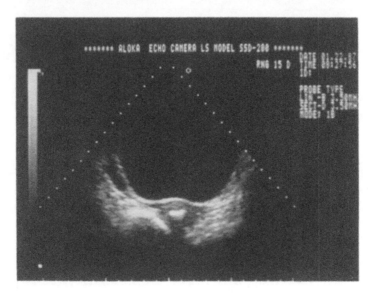

FIGURE 34.   Transverse scan of the same case.

tumor.[50] However, such sonographic features were encountered in up to 30% of histologically benign ovarian cysts; conversely, in 10 to 16% of proven malignancies, there were no sonographic signs of malignancy.[51] Therefore, a significant overlap in ultrasonic characteristics of benign and malignant tumors can be expected, and the only means by which a diagnosis can be made with certainty is by microscopic evaluation.

As far as infertile patients are concerned, the problem of ultrasound diagnosis of malignancy is less important, but because of nonspecificity of ultrasonic findings, ovarian neoplasm always should be included in differential diagnosis of adnexal masses. Various adnexal abnormalities are frequently seen in the group of infertile patients, and their sonographic demonstration is particularly helpful for diagnosing the underlying cause of infertility.

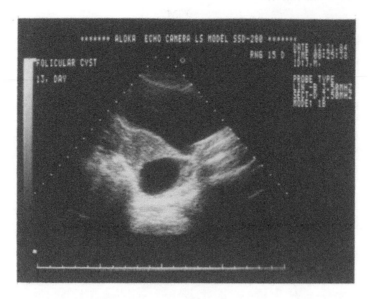

FIGURE 35. Follicular cyst in the right ovary. Normal preserved ovarian parenchyma is visible on the upper cyst pole.

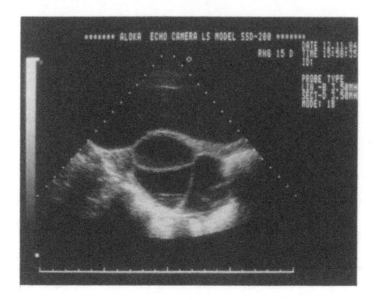

FIGURE 36. Mucinous cystadenoma exhibiting the characteristics of a complex, predominantly cystic ovarian mass.

There were several attempts to diagnose endometriosis by ultrasound. When the disease is present as a discrete pelvic mass, ultrasound is helpful to estimate localization, size, and internal consistency of the mass. The findings of a combination of cystic, complex cystic-solid, and solid masses have been described.[52] Although sonographic findings are nonspecific, a characteristic clinical history or physical examination is helpful and may promote the correct diagnosis.[53] The major problem is the diagnosis of the much more common diffuse form of the disease. That form is characterized by numerous small cysts, which can be found at almost any location within the pelvis. Because of their small size, they cannot be visualized by current equipment since they are below the resolution limits. As the largest concentration of endometriotic cysts is usually around the attachments of the uterosacral

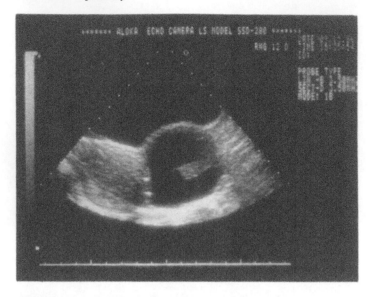

FIGURE 37.   Typical ultrasonic appearance of a dermoid cyst in a characteristic position above the uterus.

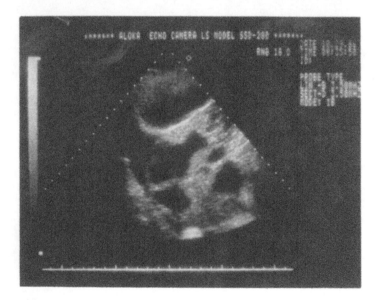

FIGURE 38.   Solid-cystic tumor with marked texture irregularities. The diagnosis of malignancy was confirmed after surgery.

ligaments to the cervix, and in the reactovaginal septum, it has been suggested that an increased background echogenicity of the pelvis may serve as an ultrasonic sign of the disease.[54] Other possibly helpful ultrasonic signs are a poor definition of the pelvic structures due to associated adhesion, and the presence of irregular cystic spaces through the myometrium, which represent concomitant adenomyosis in up to 36% of cases.[52] Unfortunately, a recent correlation of sonographic findings in 37 patients with laparoscopically proven endometriosis showed that sonography correctly identified only 10.8% of cases.[55] So, it seems that ultrasound is of limited value for diagnosis of endometriosis, particularly in cases where no large endometriomas are present (Figures 39 to 42).

Disease of the tubes is the cause of infertility in most cases. A normal fallopian tube

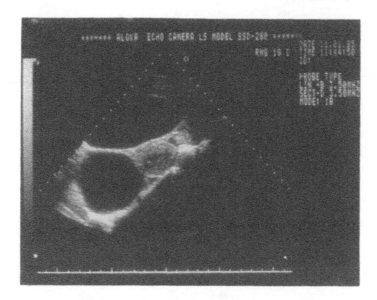

FIGURE 39. Extremely large endometriotic cyst, which is indistinguishable from a large hydrosalpinx because of its round shape, absence of internal echoes, and wall thickness.

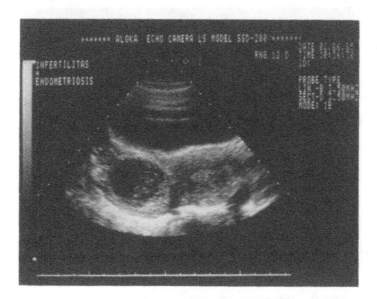

FIGURE 40. Large endometrioma (right) with pronounced internal echoes.

cannot be visualized by ultrasound, except in the presence of ascites. The tubes are most often affected by infection, and in such cases they can be visualized.

Sonographic findings in acute and chronic pelvic inflammatory disease have been reported extensively.[56-58] The earliest signs of pelvic infection are pronounced endometrial echogenicity representing endometritis, and loss of definition between the uterus, adnexa, and pelvic side walls, creating the "indefinite uterus sign". A spread into the tubes can be recognized by the demonstration of free fluid along the posterior aspect of the uterus, or the presence of pyosalpinx or tubo-ovarian abscess (Figures 43 to 46).

Several kinds of chronic inflammatory changes may occur after even one episode of acute

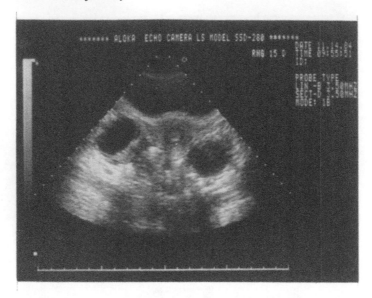

FIGURE 41.   Endometriomas in the ovaries. Note the irregular shape of the cyst and internal echoes.

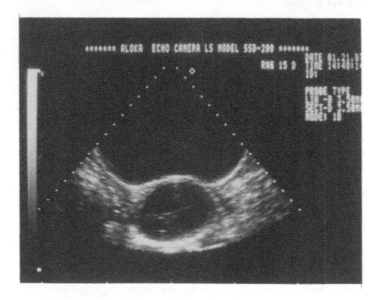

FIGURE 42.   Endometriosis. Transverse sonogram showing a large cyst on the left. The contents of the cyst are more echogenic compared to urine in the bladder.

infection, and are responsible for future infertility. Pelvic adhesions develop first, fixing pelvic structures one to another and to the adjacent bowel and omentum. If a pyosalpinx occurs, it may evolve into a hydrosalpinx in which purulent exudate is replaced by serous fluid. Pelvic sonograms may be confusing in such cases. While the adhesions themselves are invisible, they may lead to the fixation of bowel loops and omentum in the pelvis, which may in turn be mistaken for pelvic cysts and masses. The chronic residua of tubo-ovarian and pelvic abscesses such as hydrosalpinx, inflammatory cysts, and adhesions may produce complex patterns of pelvic fluid loculations, often markedly expanding the pouch of Douglas and encompassing the uterus (Figures 47 to 51).

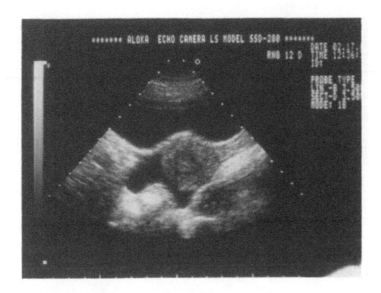

FIGURE 43. Acute pelvic infection. The transverse sonogram demonstrates a large amount of free fluid in cul-de-sac.

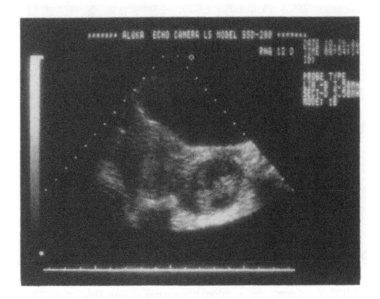

FIGURE 44. Transverse sonogram showing a large tubo-ovarian abscess on the left and above the uterus.

Without conventional clinical findings or serial sonographic changes, the ultrasound examination is not specific. An echo-free tubular pelvic structure may not represent the expected hydrosalpinx, but a dilated distal ureter. Complex residua of abscesses and inflammatory cysts may be indistinguishable from cystic neoplasms, endometriosis, or ectopic pregnancy. Functional cysts frequently coexist with chronic pelvic inflammatory disease.[59] However, the cysts usually resolve, whereas chronic pelvic inflammatory disease does not.

Normal fluid-filled bowel loops may even masquerade as abscess. The role of sonography in chronic pelvic inflammatory disease is to document the appearance of sequelae, to gauge the effectiveness of therapy, and to help to elucidate the causes of infertility.

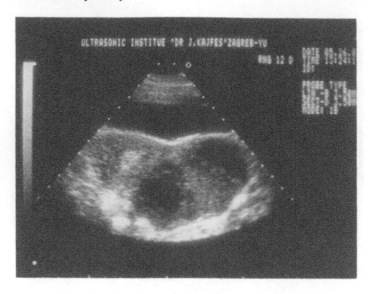

FIGURE 45.   Another example of a large left-sided tubo-ovarian abscess.

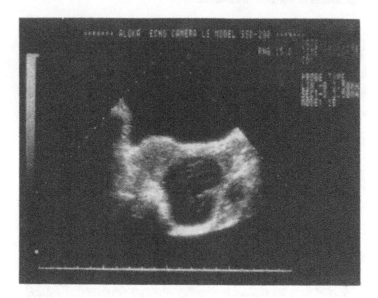

FIGURE 46.   Completely formed left tubo-ovarian abscess. Note a part of the preserved normal ovarian parenchyma in the upper left part of the complex cyst.

C. Ectopic Pregnancy

Sonography has been accepted as an important diagnostic method that is used regularly in the initial evaluation of patients with suspected ectopic pregnancy. Typical ultrasonic findings in ectopic gestation include the absence of intrauterine pregnancy, slight uterine enlargement with internal uterine echoes, and demonstration of adnexal mass and free fluid in cul-de-sac.[60] As there are numerous clinical conditions that may present the sonographic feature of ectopic gestation, such as hemorrhagic corpus luteum cysts, pelvic inflammatory disease, or endometriosis, ultrasonic findings alone allow correct positive diagnosis in approximately 75% of cases.[61] In fact, the only situation when specific ultrasonic diagnosis of ectopic pregnancy can be made is demonstration of a live embryo outside the uterus (Figures 52 to 55).

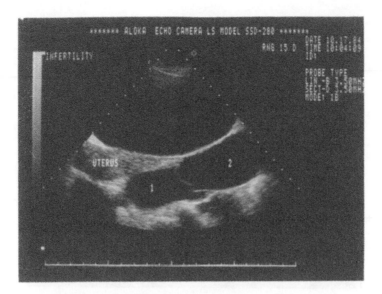

FIGURE 47. Large hydrosalpinx appearing as a bilocular cyst.

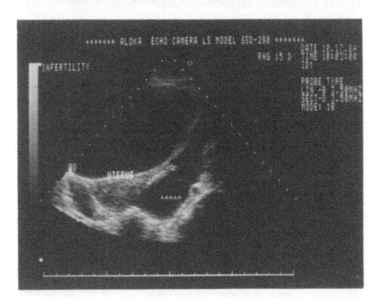

FIGURE 48. Typical fusiform shape of hydrosalpinx.

Much better results can be obtained if ultrasonic findings are interpreted together with sensitive radioimmunoassay of the β-subunit of human chorionic gonadotropin, which has been introduced recently into clinical practice. The combination of a positive serum pregnancy test and the absence of an intrauterine gestational sac on pelvic sonography accurately predicts ecotopic pregnancy in 93% of cases.[62] This approach presumes that sonography can reliably recognize the presence or absence of the intrauterine gestation. After 6 weeks of amenorrhea, the fetus can be regularly identified within the gestational sac, and such distinction is not difficult. However, particular care should be taken to differentiate intrauterine pregnancy prior to depiction of the embryonic pole from the intrauterine decidual changes. Decidual casts of an ectopic pregnancy, resembling the ultrasonic appearance of an early gestation ("pseudogestational sac"), can be seen in 20% of patients.[63] According to the recent reports, two concentric rims of decidua (the double decidual sac) can be seen in

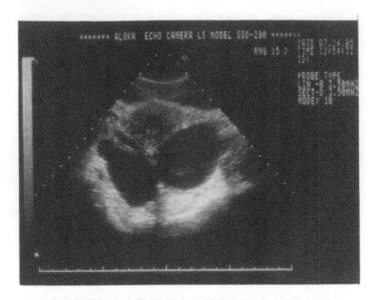

FIGURE 49.   Bilateral large hydrosalpinx in a patient suffering from infertility.

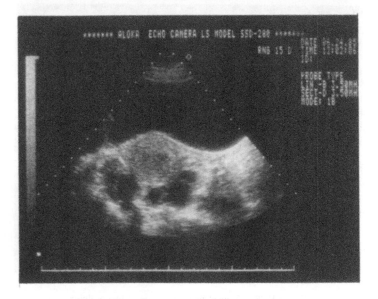

FIGURE 50.   Transverse sonogram demonstrating complex solid cystic structures in both adnexal regions and occupying the pouch of Douglas in a patient with chronic pelvic inflammation. The adhesion led to bowel loop fixation in the lesser pelvis; the loops are highly echogenic on the ultrasound scan.

98.3% of patients with early intrauterine pregnancy.[64] This finding is believed to represent the decidua capsularis around the chorionic cavity and the decidual parietalis that surrounds the decidua capsularis and developing gestational sac. The decidual cast of ectopic pregnancy, in contrast, has a single echogenic rim similar to decidua parietalis.

Although the approach described above enables an accurate diagnosis of extopic pregnancy in the vast majority of cases, there are certain situations in which these criteria may be insufficient. Cases of incomplete abortion with positive pregnancy test and nonspecific intrauterine findings present particular diagnostic problems. Moreover, recent reports have shown that the incidence of combined intra- and extrauterine pregnancy has increased from

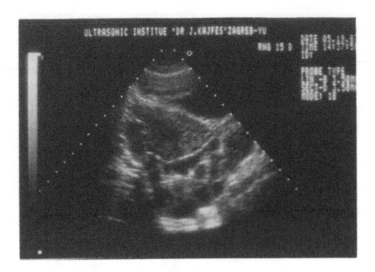

FIGURE 51.   Another example of chronic pelvic infection with bowel loops fixed within the lesser pelvis due to severe adhesion.

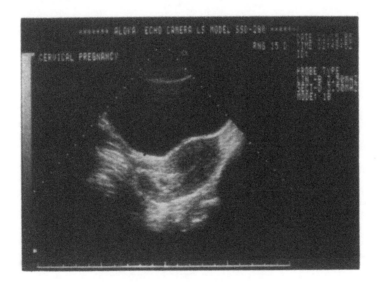

FIGURE 52.   Normal appearance of a 6-week gestational sac located in the cervical canal. A case of cervical pregnancy.

1/30,000 pregnancies to approximately 1/7,000.[65] In such cases, noncritical acceptance of evidence of an intrauterine pregnancy can alleviate suspicion of an ectopic pregnancy and cause serious danger to the patient (Figure 56).

D. Conclusion

Ultrasound, as a simple and noninvasive method, is widely and successfully used in routine clinical practice either for the demonstration of the normal anatomy of the lesser pelvis or for the detection of numerous pelvic disorders. Since ultrasonic findings are non-specific in most cases, comparison with other relevant clinical data frequently enables specific diagnosis. In the management of infertility, it is nowadays used for diagnosing the cause of

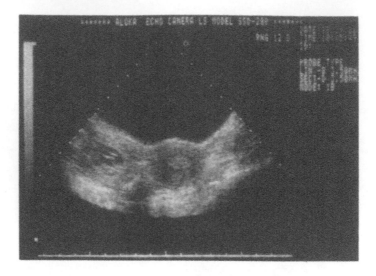

FIGURE 53.   Ectopic 8-week pregnancy with a live embryo right of the uterus in a patient with no clinical signs of ectopic pregnancy.

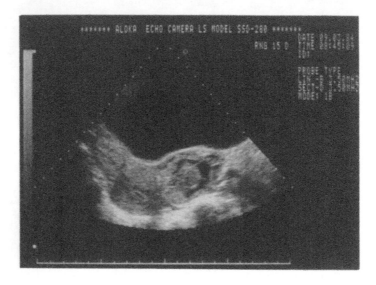

FIGURE 54.   Large hematocele on the left in a case of ectopic pregnancy.

infertility as well as for therapeutic success monitoring. At present, a single ultrasound examination of an infertile patient can provide: (1) accurate assessment of the normal anatomy of the lesser pelvis including measurement of uterine and ovarian size; (2) detection of congenital uterine anomalies; (3) diagnosis of various acquired uterine abnormalities like fibroma or adenomyosis; (4) detection of any adnexal pathology if presented as a discrete mass; (5) reliable diagnosis of an ectopic pregnancy when ultrasound findings are compared with serum β-HCG (human chorionic gonadotropin) levels; and (6) diagnosis of an early pregnancy (Table 1).

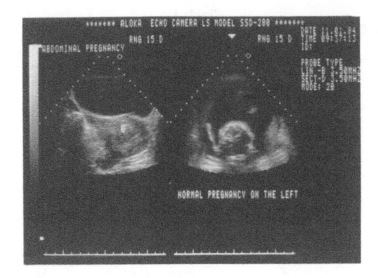

FIGURE 55.   Figure showing both the empty uterus (left) and the live fetus in a case of abdominal pregnancy (right).

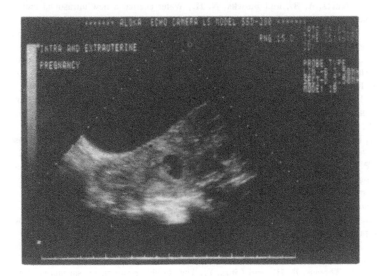

FIGURE 56.   A case of combined intra- and extrauterine pregnancy. An oblique sonogram shows two gestational sacs.

Table 1
THE CAUSES OF INFERTILITY DETECTABLE BY ULTRASOUND

Uterus
 Anomalies (aplasia, hypoplasia, uterus bicornic, etc.)
 Fibroma
 Adenomyosis
Fallopian tubes
 Pyosalpinx, hydrosalpynx
Ovaries
 Anomalies (polycystic ovaries)
 Chronic infections (tubo-ovarian abscess)
 Tumors (cystadenoma, teratoma, dermoid cyst, etc.)
Endometriosis
 Endometriosis genitalis
 Endometriosis

REFERENCES

1. **Donald, I.,** Use of ultrasonics in diagnosis of abdominal swellings, *Br. Med. J.,* 2, 1154, 1963.
2. **Rubin, C., Kurtz, A. B., and Bancks, N. H.,** Water enema: a new ultrasound technique in defining pelvic anatomy, *J. Clin. Ultrasound,* 6, 28, 1978.
3. **Bree, R. L. and Schwab, R. E.,** Contribution of mesenteric fat to unsatisfactory abdominal and pelvic ultrasonography, *Radiology,* 157, 225, 1981.
4. **Kurtz, A. B. and Rifkin, M. D.,** Normal anatomy of the female pelvis: ultrasound with computed tomography correlation, in *Principles and Practice of Ultrasonography in Obstetrics and Gynecology,* Sanders, R. C. and James, A. E., Eds., Appleton-Century-Crofts, New York, 1985, 99.
5. **Campbell, S., Goessens, L., Goswamy, R., and Whitehead, M. I.,** Real-time ultrasonography for determination of ovarian morphology and volume, *Lancet,* 1, 425, 1982.
6. **Wells, P. N. T.,** *Biomedical Ultrasonics,* Academic Press, London, 1977, 28.
7. **Kremer, H., Dobrinski, W., Mikyska, M., Baumgärtner, M., and Zöllner, N.,** Ultrasonic in vivo and in vitro studies on the nature of the ureteral jet phenomenon, *Radiology,* 142, 175, 1982.
8. **Athey, P. A.,** Uterus: abnormalities of size, shape, contour and texture, in *Ultrasound in Obstetrics and Gynecology,* Athey, P. A. and Hadlock, F. P., Eds., C. V. Mosby, St. Louis, 1985, 167.
9. **Nussbaum, A. R., Sanders, R. C., and Jones, M. D.,** Neonatal uterine morphology as seen on real-time US, *Radiology,* 160, 755, 1986.
10. **Ivarsson, S. A., Nilsson, K. O., and Persson, P. H.,** Ultrasonography of the pelvic organs in prepubertal and postpubertal girls, *Arch. Dis. Child,* 58, 352, 1983.
11. **Sample, W. F., Lippe, B. M., and Gyepes, M. T.,** Grey scale ultrasonography of the normal female pelvis, *Radiology,* 125, 477, 1977.
12. **Miller, E. I., Thomas, R. H., and Lines, P.,** The atrophic postmenopausal uterus, *J. Clin. Ultrasound,* 5, 261, 1977.
13. **Orsini, L.F., Salardi, S., Pilu, G., Bovicelli, L., and Cacciari, E.,** Pelvic organs in premenarcheal girls: real-time ultrasonography, *Radiology,* 153, 113, 1984.
14. **Fleischer,A. C., Entman, S. S., Porrath, S. A., and James, A. E.,** Sonographic evaluation of uterine malformations and disorders, in *The Principles and Practice of Ultrasonography in Obstetrics and Gynecology,* Sanders, R. C. and James, A. E., Eds., Appleton-Century-Crofts, New York, 1985, 531.
15. **Piiroinen, O.,** Ultrasonic localization of IUDs, *Acta Obstet. Gynecol. Scand.,* 51, 203, 1972.
16. **Gross, B. H. and Callen, P. W.,** Ultrasound of the uterus, in *Ultrasonography in Obstetrics and Gynecology,* Callen, P.W., Ed., W. B. Saunders, Philadelphia, 1983, 243.
17. **Callen, P. W., Demartini, W., and Filly, R.,** The central uterine cavity echo: a useful anatomic sign in the ultrasonographic evaluation of the female pelvis, *Radiology,* 131, 187, 1979.
18. **Hall, D. A., Hann, L. E., Ferrucci, J. T., Black, E. B., Braitman, B. S., Crowley, W. F., Nikrui, N., and Kalley, J. A.,** Sonographic morphology of the normal menstrual cycle, *Radiology,* 133, 185, 1979.
19. **Nakano, H., Sakamoto, C., and Koyangi, T.,** Endometrial images by ultrasound, *Acta Obstet. Gynaecol. Jpn. Engl. Ed.,* 34, 275, 1982.

20. **Sakamoto, C. and Nakano, H.,** The echogenic endometrium and alterations during menstrual cycle, *Int. J. Gynaecol. Obstet.,* 23, 7, 1982.

21. **Hackelöer, B. J.,** The role of ultrasound in female infertility management, *Ultrasound Med. Biol.,* 10, 35, 1984.

22. **Christie, A. D.,** *Ultrasound and Infertility,* Chartwel-Bratt, Bromley, England, 1981, 24.

23. **Kirkpatrick, R. H., Nikrui, N., Wittenberg, J., Hann, L., and Ferrucci, J. T.,** Gray scale ultrasound in adnexal thickening: correlation with laparoscopy, *J. Clin. Ultrasound,* 7, 115, 1979.

24. **Goswamy, R. K., Campbell, S., and Whitehead, M. I.,** Screening for ovarian cancer, *Clin. Obstet. Gynecol.,* 10, 621, 1983.

25. **Hackelöer, B. J. and Nitschke-Dabelstein, S.,** Ovarian imaging by ultrasound: an attempt to define a reference plane, *J. Clin. Ultrasound,* 8, 497, 1980.

26. **Parisi, L., Tramonti, M., and Casciano, S.,** The role of ultrasound in the study of polycystic ovarian disease, *J. Clin. Ultrasound,* 10, 167, 1982.

27. **Swanson, M., Sauerbrei, E. E., and Cooperberg, P. L.,** Medical implications of ultrasonically detected polycystic ovarian disease, *J. Clin. Ultrasound,* 9, 219, 1981.

28. **Kurjak, A. and Jurkovic, D.,** New ultrasonic technique for assessing circulation in the female pelvis, in *Recent Advances in Ultrasound Diagnosis,* Kurjak, A. and Kossoff, G., Eds., Excerpta Medica, Amsterdam, 1986, 129.

29. **Green, B.,** Pelvic ultrasonography, in *Diagnostic Ultrasound,* Sarti, D. A. and Sample, W. F., Eds., G. K. Hall, Boston, 1980, 502.

30. **Woolf, R. B. and Allen, W. B.,** Concomitant malformations: the frequent, simultaneous occurrence of congenital malformations of the reproductive and urinary tracts, *Obstet. Gynecol.,* 2, 336, 1953.

31. **Green, L. K. and Harris, R. E.,** Uterine anomalies: frequency of diagnosis and associated obstetric complications, *Obstet. Gynecol.,* 47, 427, 1976.

32. **Fried, A. M., Oliff, M., Wilson, E. A., and Whisnant, J.,** Uterine anomalies associated with renal agenesis: role of gray scale ultrasonography, *Am. J. Roentgenol.,* 131, 973, 1978.

33. **Kurtz, A. B., Wapner, R. J., Rubin, C. S., Cole-Beuglet, C., and Kendall, B.,** Bicornuate uterus: unilateral pregnancy and pelvic kidney, *J. Clin. Ultrasound,* 8, 353, 1980.

34. **Jones, T. B., Fleischer, A. C., Daniell, J. F., Lindsey, A. M., and James, A. E.,** Sonographic characteristics of congenital uterine abnormalities and associated pregnancy, *J. Clin. Ultrasound,* 8, 453, 1980.

35. **Fleischer, A. C., Entman, S. S., Burnett, L. S., and James, A. E.,** Sonographic evaluation of uterine malformations and disorders, in *The Principles and Practice of Ultrasonography in Obstetrics and Gynecology,* Sanders, R. C. and James, A. E., Eds., Appleton-Century-Crofts, New York, 1985, 531.

36. **Silverberg, S. H.,** *Principles and Practice of Surgical Pathology,* John Wiley & Sons, New York, 1983, 1323.

37. **Gross, B. H., Silver, T. M., and Jaffee, M. H.,** Sonographic features of uterine leiomyomas: analysis of 41 proven cases, *J. Ultrasound Med.,* 2, 401, 1983.

38. **Walsh, J. W., Taylor, K. J. W., Wasson, J. F., Schwartz, P. E., and Rosenfield, A. T.,** Gray-scale ultrasound in 204 proved gynecologic masses: accuracy and specific diagnostic criteria, *Radiology,* 130, 391, 1979.

39. **Von Micsky, L. L.,** Sonographic studies of uterine fibromyomata in the non-pregnant state and during gestation, in *The Principles and Practice of Ultrasonography in Obstetrics and Gynecology,* Sanders, R. C. and James, A. E., Eds., Appleton-Century-Crofts, New York, 1977, 297.

40. **Lawson, T. L. and Albarelli, J. N.,** Diagnosis of gynecologic pelvic masses by gray scale ultrasonography: analysis of specificity and accuracy, *Am. J. Roentgenol.,* 128, 1003, 1977.

41. **Requard, C. K., Mettler, F. A., and Wicks, J. D.,** Preoperative sonography of malignant ovarian noeplasms, *Am. J. Roentgenol.,* 137, 79, 1981.

42. **Fleischer, A. C., James, A. E., Millis, J. B., and Julian, C.,** Differential diagnosis of pelvic masses by gray-scale sonography, *Am. J. Roentgenol.,* 131, 469, 1978.

43. **Guttman, P. H.,** In search of the elusive benign cystic ovarian teratoma: application of the ultrasound "tip of the iceberg" sign, *J. Clin. Ultrasound,* 5, 403, 1976.

44. **Quinn, S. F., Erickson, S., and Black, W. C.,** Cystic ovarian teratomas: the sonographic appearance of the dermoid plug, *Radiology,* 155, 477, 1985.

45. **Sandler, M. A., Silver, T. M., and Karo, J. J.,** Gray-scale features of ovarian teratoma, *Radiology,* 131, 705, 1979.

46. **Laing, F. C., Van Dalsem, V. F., Marks, W. M., Barton, J. L., and Martinez, D. A.,** Dermoid cysts of the ovary: their ultrasonographic appearance, *Obstet. Gynecol.,* 57, 99, 1981.

47. **Takeuchi, H.,** Ultrasonic diagnosis of gynecological tumors, in *Ultrasonic Differential Diagnosis of Tumors,* Kossoff, G. and Fukuda, M., Eds., Igaku-Shoin, Tokyo, 1984, 251.

48. **Fleischer, A. C., Entman, S. S., Burnett, L. S., and James, A. E.,** Principles of differential diagnosis of pelvic masses by sonography, in *The Principles and Practice of Ultrasonography in Obstetrics and Gynecology,* Sanders, R. C. and James, A. E., Eds., Appleton-Century-Crofts, New York, 1985, 457.
49. **Meine, H. B., Farrant, P., and Guha, T.,** Distinction of benign from malignant ovarian cysts by ultrasound, *Br. J. Obstet. Gynecol.,* 85, 893, 1978.
50. **Moyle, J. W.,** Sonography of ovarian tumors: predictability of tumor type, *Am. J. Roentgenol.,* 141, 985, 1983.
51. **Morley, P. M. and Barnett, E.,** The ovarian mass, in *The Principles and Practice of Ultrasonography in Obstetrics and Gynecology,* Sanders, R. C. and James, A. E., Eds., Appleton-Century-Crofts, New York, 1985, 473.
52. **Walsh, J. W., Taylor, K. J. W., and Rosenfield, A. T.,** Gray scale ultrasonography in the diagnosis of endometriosis and adenomyosis, *Am. J. Roentgenol.,* 132, 87, 1979.
53. **Coleman, B. G., Arger, P. H., and Mulhern, C. B.,** Endometriosis: clinical and ultrasonic correlation, *Am. J. Roentgenol.,* 132, 747, 1979.
54. **Birnholz, J. C.,** Endometriosis and inflammatory disease, *Semin. Ultrasound,* 4, 184, 1983.
55. **Friedman, H., Vogelzang, R. L., Mendelson, E. B., Nieman, H. L., and Cohen, M.,** Endometriosis detection by US with laparoscopic correlation, *Radiology,* 157, 217, 1985.
56. **Urich, P. C. and Sanders, R. C.,** Ultrasonic characteristics of pelvic inflammatory masses, *J. Clin. Ultrasound,* 4, 199, 1976.
57. **Bowie, J. D.,** Ultrasound of gynecologic pelvic masses: the indefinite uterus sign and other patterns associated with diagnostic error, *J. Clin. Ultrasound,* 5, 323, 1977.
58. **Athey, P. A.,** Uterus: abnormalities of size, shape, contour and texture, in *Ultrasound in Obstetrics and Gynecology,* Athey, P. A. and Hadlock, F. P., Eds., C. V. Mosby, St. Louis, 1985, 167.
59. **Hamilton, C. J. C. M., Evers, J. L. H., and Hoogland, H. J.,** Ovulatory disorders and inflammatory adnexal damage: a neglected cause of the failure of fertility microsurgery, *Br. J. Obstet. Gynaecol.,* 93, 282, 1986.
60. **Lawson, T. L.,** Ectopic pregnancy: criteria and accuracy of ultrasonic diagnosis, *Am. J. Roentgenol.,* 131, 153, 1978.
61. **Brown, T. W., Filly, R. A., Laing, F. C., and Barton, J.,** Analysis of ultrasonographic criteria in the evaluation of ectopic pregnancy, *Am. J. Roentgenol.,* 131, 967, 1978.
62. **Weckstein, L. N., Boucher, A. R., and Tucker, H.,** Accurate diagnosis of early ectopic pregnancy, *Obstet. Gynecol.,* 65, 393, 1985.
63. **Marks, W. M.,** The decidual cast of ectopic pregnancy: a confusing ultrasonographic appearance, *Radiology,* 133, 451, 1979.
64. **Nyberg, D., Laing, F., and Filly, F.,** Ultrasonic differentiation of the gestational sac of early intrauterine pregnancy from the pseudogestational sac of ectopic pregnancy, *Radiology,* 146, 755, 1983.
65. **Reece, E. A., Petrie, R. H., Sirmans, M. F., Finster, M., and Todd, W. D.,** Combined intrauterine and extrauterine gestations: a review, *Am. J. Obstet. Gynecol.,* 146, 323, 1983.

Chapter 4

ULTRASONIC MONITORING OF FOLLICULAR GROWTH AND OVULATION IN SPONTANEOUS AND STIMULATED CYCLES

Asim Kurjak and Davor Jurkovic

TABLE OF CONTENTS

I. INTRODUCTION

Detection and accurate prediction of ovulation are two of the main problems in the management of female infertility. The availability of accurate laboratory methods for determining peripheral hormone levels has improved substantially the accuracy of the ovulation prediction. These methods have supplemented time-honored clinical observations where the patient's end-organ responses to the hormonal changes are assessed (i.e., the basal body temperature, cervical score, and vaginal cytology). All these methods are designed to assess the hormonal events associated with the follicular development and ovum release, and are therefore indirect.

Recently, ultrasound has provided a new method for the evaluation of ovarian function, with reference to both follicular development and corpus luteum function. Kratochwil et al.[1] first described and illustrated in 1972 that ovaries could be visualized by ultrasound and that follicles could also be identified. Following those initial observations, the first systematic investigations with ultrasonic demonstration of follicular development during the spontaneous and stimulated cycles were performed in 1977.[2] Since then, numerous authors have confirmed the initial observations that ultrasound provides a simple and noninvasive insight into physiological changes during the menstrual cycle, and accurate and reproducible studies of follicular size during the late follicular phase.[3-5]

II. EXAMINATION TECHNIQUE

The technique employed for the ultrasound monitoring of follicular growth is more or less the same as for the routine scanning of gynecological patients. The basic prerequisite for clear visualization of anatomical details within the lesser pelvis is an optimal bladder filling. As the examinations are performed serially for several days, it is of particular importance that each patient acquire her own bladder regime. This can be achieved easily if scanning is performed daily and always at the same time. Thus, after a few days the patients are able to get used to the inconvenient sense of a full bladder and to fill the bladder spontaneously, alleviating the need to use diuretics.

Static B-mode gray-scale scanners were for a long time considered to provide the best visualization of anatomical details within the lesser pelvis, but recent improvements in real-time mechanical sector resolution capabilities bring up the fact that their imaging capabilities gradually match those of static machines. Examinations with real-time sector probes are much more simple and less time consuming when compared with the static machines, and the ultrasonic findings are less operator dependent. These obvious advantages of real-time machines have made them the currently preferred mode of pelvic sonographic imaging (Figure 1).

With the patient lying supine, the probe is placed suprapubically, and parallel transverse and longitudinal scans are employed to define uterine and ovarian position. After these procedures, oblique scans are performed for better delineation of each particular structure. By using this technique, one can easily visualize ovaries in more than 99% of patients being examined.[6] Extreme variability of ovarian position can occasionally pose certain difficulties during examination, which are almost regularly overcome by a good scanning technique. There also is the possibility of visualizing pelvic vessels, which then may be used as a reference plan to detect the ovarian position.[7] Ovarian vessels reach the ovary through the infundibulopelvic ligament, and their position to the ovaries is considerably constant. Unfortunately, ovarian vessels are very thin structures and are not clearly seen in the majority of cases, which makes their use for this purpose uncertain. Internal iliac artery and vein typically pass lateral and posterior to the ovaries and due to their large diameter, are regularly seen. However, if the ovaries are atypically located, this is not the case, and the use of iliac vessels as a reference plan is not justifiable.[8]

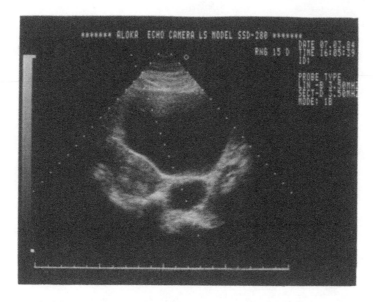

FIGURE 1. Transverse B-mode real-time scan showing a normal uterus (UT) and both ovaries. The right ovary (OV) is of ovoid shape and displays slightly lower echogenicity compared to the uterus. The left ovary contains a developing follicle (FOL) that appears as a small and ovoid cystic structure with well-defined walls and clear fluid within.

Table 1
BASIC CHARACTERISTICS
OF THE METHOD OF
SONOGRAPHIC
FOLLICULAR GROWTH
AND OVULATION
MONITORING

3- to 5-MHz real-time sector probe
Full bladder technique
Daily examinations from days 9 and 10
All examinations by the same observer

Monitoring of follicular growth and ovulation by ultrasound should be started on day 9 or 10 of a regular 28-d menstrual cycle. Depending on the cycle length, serial examinations may be attempted a few days earlier or later. The best results could be achieved if all examinations in each particular patient are performed by the same observer (Table 1; Figure 2).

III. SPONTANEOUS CYCLES

In each menstrual cycle, only one follicle from the cohort of 15 to 20 small antral follicles present in the ovaries during the late luteal phase of the previous cycle is selected and destined to reach full maturity. The exact mechanism of selection is not completely understood, but it seems that it depends mostly on the dominant follicle inherent capability of estrogen synthesis.[9,10] Because of its significantly larger amount of granulosa cells and higher aromatase activity, the precursor follicle has the lowest requirement for the sustained follicle-stimulating hormone (FSH) stimulation. This enables its further development in spite of markedly decreased FSH values during the late luteal and early follicular phase of the cycle.

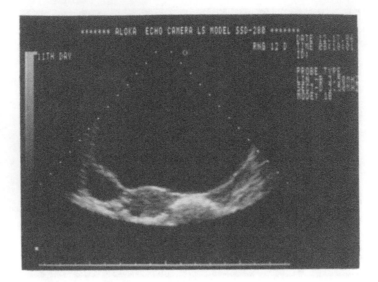

FIGURE 2.   Real-time sector scan of the mature preovulatory follicle in the right ovary on day 11 of the menstrual cycle.

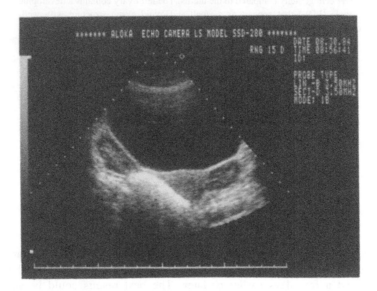

FIGURE 3.   Transverse sonogram of the uterus and both ovaries in the post-menstrual phase of the cycle. Small cysts affecting ovarian texture homogenicity can always be seen. The dominant follicle cannot be distinguished from the other antral follicles in this phase of the cycle.

Increased estrogen production by the precursor follicle provides negative feedback on pituitary FSH production and sustains low levels of FSH in peripheral blood. Thus, FSH levels are below the threshold requirements of other antral follicles that undergo atresia.

Although the process of selection is completed in the early follicular phase of the cycle, by the immediate postmenstrual scanning of the ovaries it is not possible to distinguish the precursor follicle from the other antral follicles present in the ovaries. A typical ultrasonic finding in that period of the cycle is the presence of five to ten small cystic structures within the ovaries representing the antral follicle which do not differ in their size or morphological appearance (Figure 3).[13]

From 3 to 5 d before ovulation, i.e., days 8 to 10 of a regular 28-d cycle, the dominant follicle can be identified as an anechoic cystic structure with well-defined borders, measuring 8 to 10 mm in size, and being significantly larger than other follicles still present within the ovaries. During the next several days the preovulatory follicle undergoes fast growth, and a day before ovulation, it reaches a diameter of 20 mm (Figures 4 to 6).[14,15]

The basic ultrasonic parameter for the assessment of follicular maturation is the diameter of the dominant follicle. The size of the follicle is measured by means of an in-built digital caliper system. By positioning two bright calipers on the inner walls of the follicle, as it would be seen on the frozen image on the screen, the diameter is automatically displayed (Figure 7). Even though the basic technique of the measurement is the same, there are significant differences in size of the preovulatory follicle between various reports (Table 2; Graph 1). This can be attributed partly to the differences among the used equipment and experience, but the major source of the wide range of values lies in the number of planes in which the measurements were performed. Early reports were based on either single maximal or two- or three-diameter measurements. Nowadays, most authors are estimating the follicle size by calculating the mean diameter from linear measurements taken in three orthogonal planes.[16] In view of the fact that the shape of the follicle is rarely round, but more commonly is ovoid or elongated, this approach gives the most reliable information about actual follicular size. By performing measurement of three diameters, one can easily calculate the volume of the follicular fluid. It does not represent an improvement over the mean diameter estimation for the assessment of follicular growth, but it can be useful in certain situations (e.g., before aspiration of follicular fluid for *in vitro* fertilization).

The daily growth rate of the preovulatory follicle is between 2 to 3 mm and parallels rising estradiol levels. On the basis of previous studies which showed that more than 90% of circulating estradiol is produced by the preovulatory follicle,[17] Hackelöer et al.[18] have compared ultrasonic follicular measurements with endocrinological parameters of follicular growth and maturity. Their results showed that there was a clear-cut correlation between the diameter of the growing follicle and peripheral estradiol levels estimated by radioimmunoassay, when mean values of either both parameters or paired data were analyzed for days −5 to 0. Synchronous analysis of the leutinizing hormone (LH) profile in the same study showed a regular coincidence of midcycle LH surge with the maximal diameter of the preovulatory follicle. These data clearly show that on the basis of morphological studies of the growing follicle, it is possible to collect information about its functional capability. It could be helpful for interpreting the peripheral target organ and plasma steroid level changes, particularly in cases of abnormal cycles, which are discussed later (Graph 2).

The most common indication for the ovarian scanning during the spontaneous cycles is better prediction of ovulation in patients who are undergoing artificial insemination (Table 3). However, accurate prediction and detection of ovulation carry critical importance in the success of this procedure. Although the ultrasound scanning is particularly reliable for the detection of ovulation, prediction of ovulation, based on the diameter of the dominant follicle alone, is not sufficiently accurate.[19] As previously reported, the mean diameter of the preovulatory follicle a day before ovulation is about 20 mm, but the range of values is wide, between 16 to 25 mm. For this reason, several authors have tried to define minor morphological changes in the appearance of the preovulatory follicle which are suggestive of imminent ovulation.

It is well documented that midcycle LH surge induces numerous morphological changes in the preovulatory follicle. LH surge is triggered by high estradiol levels above 500 pmol/l which are sustained for 2 to 3 d. Specific organization of the synthesis and secretion of LH in the pituitary gonadotropes, which presumes the presence of two hormone pools, is most probably a critical event, which enables a qualitative shift from the negative feedback to the positive one.[20,21]

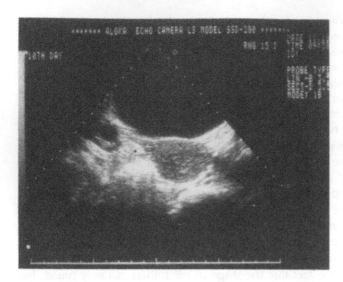

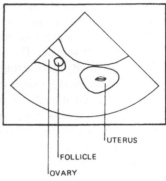

FIGURE 4.

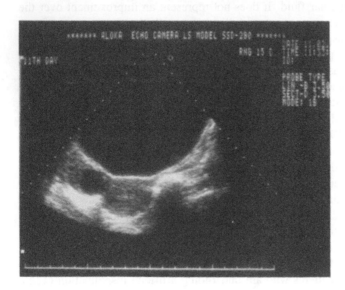

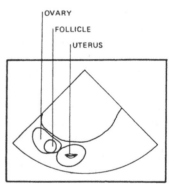

FIGURE 5.

FIGURES 4 to 6   Illustrations of the growth of the preovulatory follicle in the late follicular phase of the cycle as seen on serial daily ultrasound examinations.

The most important changes in the preovulatory follicle include the shift of steroidogenesis in granulosa cells from estrogen to progesterone, luteinization of granulosa cells, and initiation of the final oocyte maturation. This is accompanied by dissociation of the cumulus oophorus and separation of granulosa and theca layers.[22] Some of these features can be recognized by ultrasound.

Bomsel-Helmreich et al.[23] obtained clear evidence that the ultrasonic appearance of the triangular intrafollicular echogenic structure, regularly seen adjacent to the inner wall of the follicle, represents the dissociated cumulus oophorus. According to their results, echo of

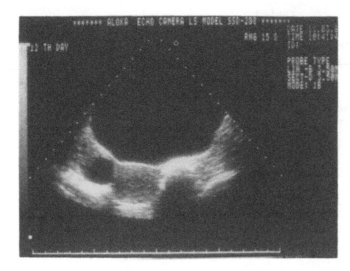

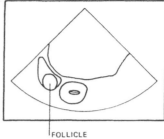

FIGURE 6.

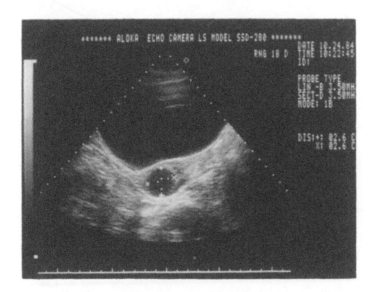

FIGURE 7. Oblique scan through the right ovary with an illustration of the ovarian follicle measurement technique. Diameter of the follicle should be measured in three orthogonal planes by placing the calipers on the inner wall of the follicle.

the cumulus oophorus can be demonstrated in the preovulatory follicle only after its dissociation, and therefore can be used as a reliable sign that LH surge has already occurred. Although this finding indicates forthcoming ovulation, its use in the assessment of the ovarian function is limited by the relatively low visualization rate of 15 to 20% of cases.[24] There are a few reports that claim a much higher visualization rate of the cumulus oophorus, but to obtain such results, exceptionally good equipment, meticulous examination of the entire follicular surface, and extensive experience are required (Figure 8).[25]

The presence of a well-defined echo of the cumulus oophorus allows accurate prediction of ovulation within the next 24 h, but a negative finding does not imply its absence and should be critically accepted.

Table 2
THE SIZE OF THE
PREOVULATORY FOLLICLE IN
NORMAL SPONTANEOUS
CYCLES

No. of monitored cycles	Mean values (mm)	Ref.
15	19.8	18
18	27.0	69
7	12.8	70
20	10.0	71
25	20.6	15
23	20.7	72
30	20.5	25
21	23.1	11

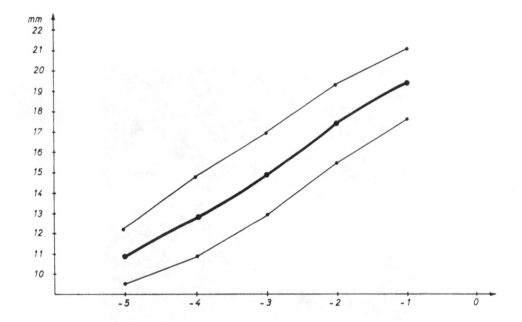

GRAPH 1. Average diameter of the dominant follicle from days −5 to −1. Day 0 = ovulation; mean ± SD; N = 50.

Another very consistent ultrasonic feature in the preovulatory follicle is related to the morphology of the follicular wall, and this was first reported by Picker et al.[26] in 1983. It has been described as a line of decreased echogenicity around the follicle and may be seen within 24 h before ovulation. The finding was explained by the histological studies of the preovulatory follicle after LH surge, which showed edematous thecal tissue and separation of granulosa and theca cell layers. As ovulation approaches, separation is progressive and causes folding of the granulosa cell layer which can be demonstrated sonographically as a crenation of the follicle wall. Massive separation and folding of the granulosa occur just a few hours before ovulation, and for that reason it is rarely seen with a usual one-per-day frequency of examinations (Figure 9).[26]

Numerous biochemical changes that are also induced in the preovulatory follicle by midcycle LH surge result with the rupture of the preovulatory follicle 30 to 36 h later.

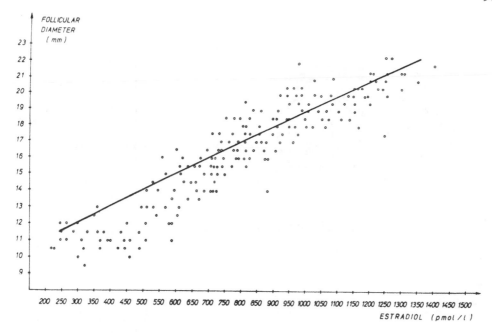

GRAPH 2. Linear correlation between the diameter of the dominant follicle and plasma estradiol levels from days −5 to −1 relative to the day of ultrasonically observed ovulation. r = 0.794; p <0.01; N = 189.

Table 3
THE ROLE OF ULTRASOUND
IN SPONTANEOUS CYCLE
ASSESSMENT

Visualization of pelvic anatomy
Reproducible studies of follicular growth
Accurate diagnosis of ovulation
Improved prediction of ovulation
Detection of abnormal cycles

Increased progesterone and cAMP synthesis activate in some way the proteolytic enzymes collagenase and plasmin, resulting in the digestion of collagen in the follicular wall and an increase in its distensibility. Increased prostaglandin synthesis seems to play a pivotal role in the mechanism of follicular rupture. If prostaglandin synthesis inhibitors are administered to experimental animals, the mature preovulatory follicle fails to rupture in spite of the normal midcycle LH surge.[27] The previous hypothesis that the follicle ruptures because of high preovulatory pressure was abandoned on the basis of direct measurements. They showed low pressure before ovulation and this is in accordance with laparoscopic visualization of gentle, rather than explosive, rupture of the stigma.[28,29]

The process of ovulation and follicular rupture also has been demonstrated by ultrasound.[30] There were no significant changes in either the size or morphology of the follicle before its sudden decrease in size, which denotes escape of follicular fluid in the periovarian region. It took between 7 to 35 min until complete collapse of the follicle. As early as 1 h after rupture, the corpus hemorrhagicum may be visualized. Sonographically demonstrated, the early corpus luteum may have varying appearance and this occasionally can cause difficulties in diagnosis of ovulation. The most common feature includes complete collapse of the follicle and the presence of a small residual cyst with thick walls. It is usually filled with

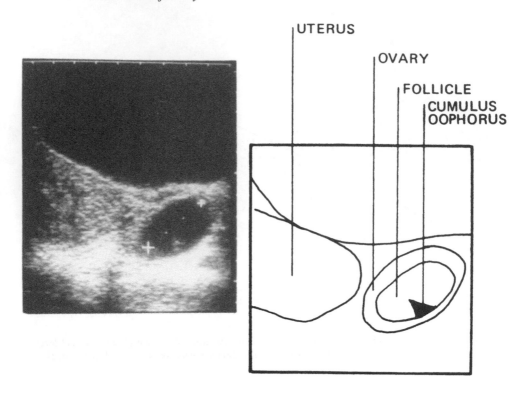

FIGURE 8.   Real-time scan of the mature preovulatory follicle demonstrates a triangular echo of the cumulus oophorus.

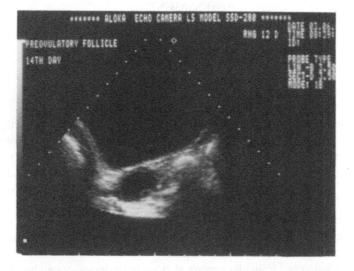

FIGURE 9.   Massive separation of the granulosa cells in the mature preovulatory follicle is seen as a thin echogenic line close to the posterior follicle wall.

echogenic blood clots. In such cases, diagnosis of ovulation is relatively simple and reliable. In about 20% of cases, the follicle is almost the same or slightly decreased in size. It loses its tense appearance and is also filled with echogenic material. This represents a reaccumulation of the fluid and blood within the ruptured follicle and is accepted as clear ultrasonic

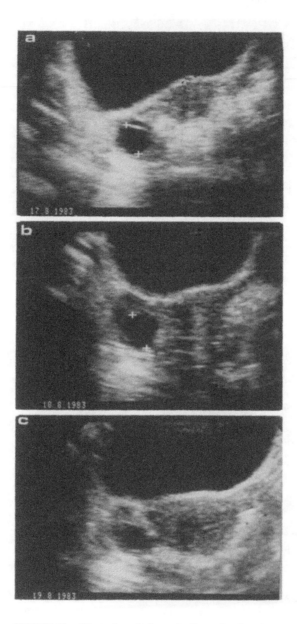

FIGURE 10. Illustration of ultrasonic diagnosis of ovulation after serial daily scanning. The dominant follicle is seen in the right ovary on day 12 of the cycle. (a) On the following day, there is an obvious increase in the follicular size, and mean diameter reached 19 mm. (b) On day 14, there is a significant change in the appearance of the follicle. Its size is markedly reduced, the walls are thick, and it is partly filled with an echogenic material. (c) This represents the typical ultrasonic signs of ovulation and early corpus luteum formation.

evidence of ovulation as well. The most controversial finding is the presence of a cyst of the same or even larger size with tense walls and some internal echoes. This finding is highly suggestive of defective ovulation and is discussed in detail later (Figures 10 and 11).

Although the main morphological changes related to the menstrual cycle concern the ovaries, important findings are also demonstrated in the pouch of Douglas and uterine mucosa.

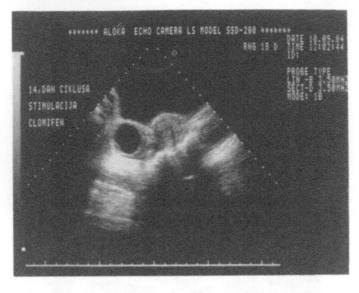

A

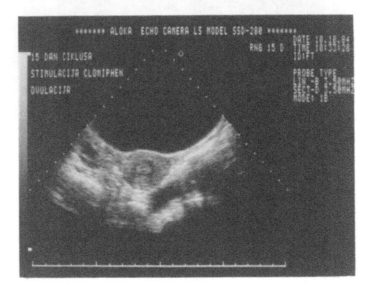

B

FIGURE 11. Another example of ultrasonic diagnosis of ovulation. The mature follicle that was clearly defined in the right ovary on day 14 of the cycle (A) almost completely disappeared when examination was repeated on the following day (B).

Peritoneal fluid does not increase much in quantity during the follicular phase, but during the luteal phase its volume increases to 10 to 30 ml. The peritoneal fluid is above all an exudation product from the turgid vessels of a functioning ovary. This is confirmed by the presence of a particularly low quantity of peritoneal fluid in women using contraceptive pills and in menopausal women.

An abrupt increase in the amount of peritoneal fluid may be sonographically documented in 25% of patients after ovulation.[30] However, this finding does not necessarily imply that

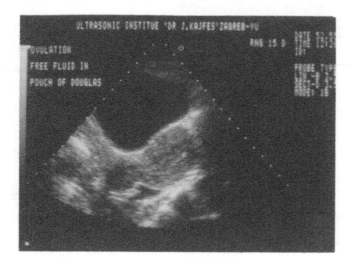

FIGURE 12.   Longitudinal scan showing free fluid in the pouch of Douglas after ovulation.

ovulation has occurred, but may be useful as an indirect and additional sign that ovulation has taken place (Figure 12).

In the immediate postmenstrual phase, the endometrium is seen as a thin, highly echoic linear echo. During the second week of the proliferative phase, it becomes gradually thicker, and is characterized by a thin and well-defined boundary within the myometrium. A marked linear middle echo represents the attached superficial endometrial layers. The endometrium is hypoechoic compared to the echogenicity of the myometrium. This can be explained by the presence of edematous fluid, which separates the stroma cells of the superficial layer (Figures 13 to 15).

In the preovulatory phase of the cycle, the endometrium is 3.5 to 7 mm thick as measured by ultrasound. A day before ovulation, there is an obvious increase in its echogenicity, particularly in the basal portions. Middle echo is less pronounced, but still present (Figures 16 and 17).[31]

In the midluteal phase, the endometrium is thick and homogeneous. The endometrial surfaces do not adhere to each other as in the proliferative phase, and the linear echo is, therefore, lost. The endometrium is highly echogenic and clearly visible (Figure 18).[32]

These ultrasonically obtained data about the morphological characteristics of endometrium correspond well to the classic histological descriptions. The accuracy of endometrial thickness measurement by ultrasound has been proved comparing the ultrasonically and histologically estimated endometrial size, which showed an excellent correlation.[33]

The characteristic ultrasonic appearance of the preovulatory endometrium resembles the ultrasonic finding of an early gestational sac, well known as the "ovulation ring". For a long time, it has served as an additional parameter for detection of ovulation (Figure 19).[8]

We have recently correlated morphological characteristics of the endometrium during the normal spontaneous cycles, including its thickness and echogenicity, to the peripheral plasma steroid hormone levels. In the proliferative phase of the cycle, there was significant correlation between estradiol levels and endometrial thickness. The increased echogenicity of the endometrium in the preovulatory phase was regularly associated with a significant increase of progesterone levels above baseline values. Increased echogenicity of the endometrium may be explained by a fast increase in glycogen content. Glycogen is a characteristic substance of secretory endometrium and can be found in the endometrial cells as early as

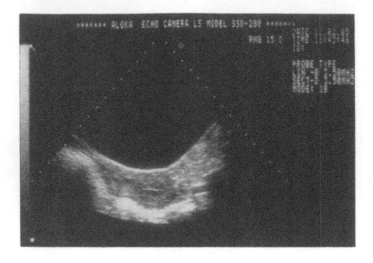

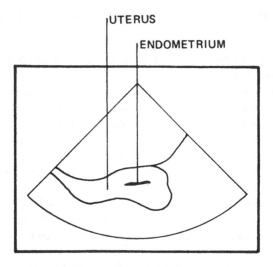

FIGURE 13.   Longitudinal sonogram of the uterus in the early proliferative phase of the cycle showing a strong uterine cavity echo. This strong
echo represents the thin endometrium with attached superficial layers and
can be seen regularly in early proliferation.

2 h after progesterone administration to the castrated patient.[34] Sonographic studies have
demonstrated that glycogen is a strongly echogenic substance, contributing primarily to the
echogenicity of the choroid plexus in second-trimester fetuses and of the small bowel in
children and adults.[35,36]

Assessment of endometrial changes during ultrasound monitoring of follicular growth
provides additional data about the functional capability of the growing follicle. It could be
particularly useful for better prediction of ovulation, fast and simple orientation about the
phase of the menstrual cycle, and detection of certain cycle abnormalities (Graph 3).

During the luteal phase of the cycle, the corpus luteum can be seen in approximately 60%
of patients. However, the corpus luteum morphology has low specificity, and demonstration
of its characteristics is only of academic interest because it does not offer any relevant clinical
information.

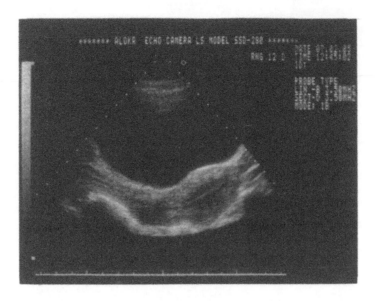

FIGURE 14.   Transverse sonogram showing the endometrium in the early proliferative phase.

IV. ABNORMAL CYCLES

Nowadays, ultrasound is widely used in the management of infertile patients. Expansion of the use of sonography in this field can be easily explained by its noninvasiveness and possibility to give numerous relevant clinical data in an extremely short time. At present, a single ultrasound examination can provide an accurate assessment of the normal anatomy of the lesser pelvis, including measurement of uterine and ovarian size, diagnosis of various congenital anomalies, and detection of any pelvic pathology presented as a discrete mass. However, the usefulness of ultrasound for the detection of ovulation disorders has been recognized just recently, following introduction of follicular growth and ovulation monitoring into routine clinical practice.

Obviously, in the group of patients suffering from chronic anovulation, due to either peripheral or central hypothalamic-pituitary endocrine disorders, this method can be used only for evaluation of efficiency and side effects of applied therapy. As far as this group of patients is concerned, ultrasound remains particularly helpful for diagnosing polycystic ovarian disease. This is a complex endocrinological disorder characterized by bilateral symmetrical ovarian enlargement and microcystic changes in their internal structure. It always results in chronic anovulation and is associated with numerous clinical signs: hirsutism, obesity, menstrual irregularities, and infertility.

Polycystic ovarian disease is clinically diagnosed by the analysis of hormonal levels, which are, however, extremely variable and not disturbed exclusively by the presence of ovarian disease. Ultrasound demonstration of ovarian enlargement and characteristic morphological appearance are important for accurate diagnosis of polycystic ovarian disease. A typical ultrasonic appearance of this condition is a bilateral ovarian enlargement with numerous small cysts that range from 2 to 6 mm in size. Although ovarian enlargement has been clearly demonstrated by using static equipment, intraovarian cysts could be seen more clearly by applying real-time machines. In 20% of patients, a polycystic pattern cannot be demonstrated, but the ovaries appear hypoechoic and many thick echoes arranged along parallel lines can be seen (Figures 20 and 21).[37,38]

The ultrasonic appearance of polycystic ovaries is associated with the disease in 75 to

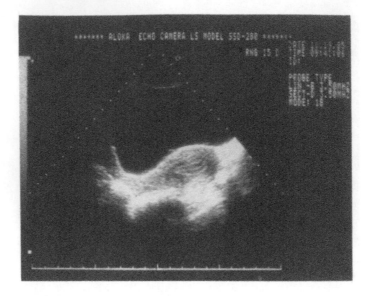

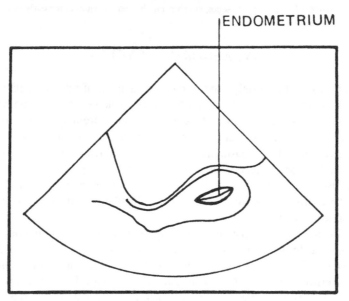

FIGURE 15. The endometrium in the late proliferative phase. The endometrium is hypoechoic compared to the myometrium and its boundary within the latter is well defined. The central echo of the attached superficial layers is also clearly visible.

96% of cases.[39,40] However, in 25 to 29% of cases, polycystic ovarian disease does not cause ovarian enlargement, and ultrasonic demonstration of normal-sized ovaries does not necessarily imply the absence of the disease. The accuracy of ultrasonic diagnosis of the disease may be improved if the criteria, which include the assessment of ovarian stroma, are included in the diagnosis. According to Franks et al.,[41] the increased stroma is an important feature since it helps to distinguish the polycystic ovaries from the multifollicular appearance. These may be seen as a temporary feature of normal pubertal development, or in weight-loss amenorrhea. Such multicystic ovaries do not contain increased stroma and appear to be normal ovaries that are receiving abnormal gonadotrophin stimulation.

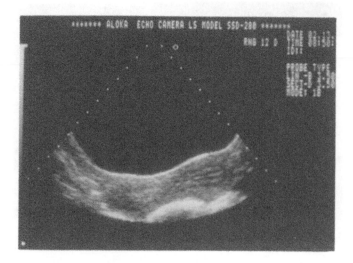

FIGURE 16. Typical appearance of the preovulatory endometrium exhibiting increased basal layer echogenicity.

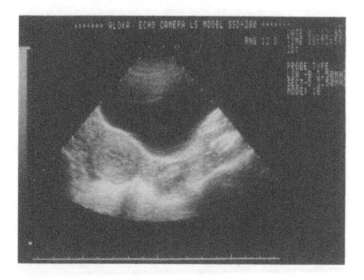

FIGURE 17. Preovulatory endometrium appearance as demonstrated on the longitudinal scan.

A particularly interesting part of the ultrasound assessment of spontaneous cycles is the detection of abnormal follicular growth or disturbed ovulation in apparently normal cycles. Wide use of sonographic follicular monitoring has confirmed the previous hypothesis that ovulation abnormalities may be found in patients with normal cycle length and biphasic basal body temperature curve, as well as in certain cases with normal gonadotrophin and steroid hormone levels throughout the menstrual cycle. (Figure 22).

Ultrasound detection of disturbed ovulation in such cases is based on well-defined morphological criteria for normal follicular growth and ovulation in comparison to radioimmunoassay of pituitary and ovarian hormones in peripheral blood. Even in their early report, which actually established the important role of sonography for the studies of ovarian function, Hackelöer et al.[18] described 3 cases of apparently abnormal follicular maturation,

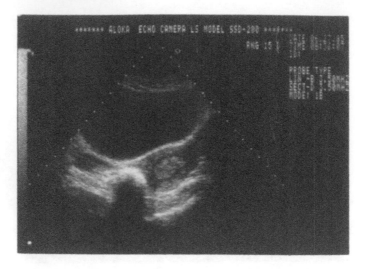

FIGURE 18. Echogenic endometrium in the secretory phase. The endometrium is thick and the central echo is lost.

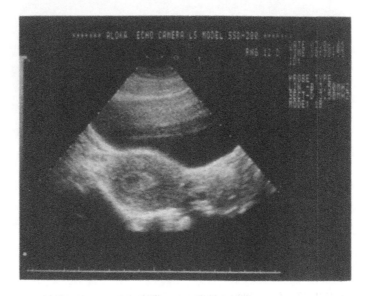

FIGURE 19. Ultrasonic demonstration of the "ovulation ring" resembling an early intrauterine pregnancy appearance.

confirmed by hormone assays, in a group of 15 healthy volunteers. The significance of sonographically observed follicle maturation and ovulation abnormalities has been confirmed in numerous subsequent reports. Polan et al.[42] have found various cycle abnormalities in 5 of 14 women (38%) suffering from secondary infertility. The common ultrasonic finding in this group of patients was demonstration of a significantly smaller size of the preovulatory follicle with asynchronicity between its morphological characteristics and serum levels of ovarian steroids and LH. Elevated progesterone levels in the luteal phase and biphasic basal body temperature curve were seen in all patients with abnormal ultrasonic findings. Based on these results, the authors have pointed out an inadequacy of standard criteria for the ovulatory cycle. This can partly explain the failure of achieving pregnancy in patients who apparently respond well to ovarian stimulation or patients in whom numerous unsuccessful artificial inseminations were attempted.[42]

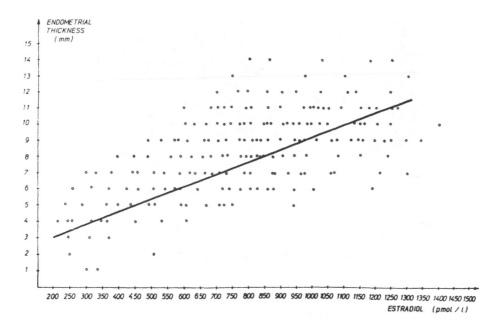

GRAPH 3. Graph illustrating the linear correlation between the thickness of the endometrium as measured by ultrasound, and peripheral plasma estradiol levels from days −5 to −1 as related to the day of ovulation. r = 0.53; p <0.01; N = 189.

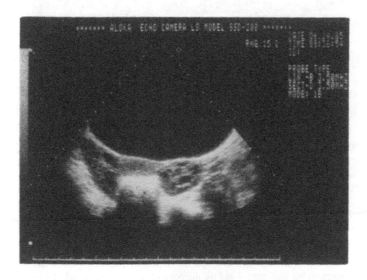

FIGURE 20. Transverse sonogram of a patient with amenorrhea and hirsutism. Both ovaries are enlarged and polycystic. The uterus is small and hypoplastic.

A similar conclusion could be drawn from the report of Coutts et al.,[43] who have found cycle abnormalities in 13 of 25 investigated cycles in a group of patients with unexplained infertility. A regular finding in the luteal phase of abnormal cycles was the presence of an intraovarian cyst with acoustic characteristics markedly different from the normal corpus luteum. Luteal progesterone levels were significantly lower compared to the normal ovulatory cycles.

Among the ultrasonically detectable cycle abnormalities, the diagnosis of luteinized un-

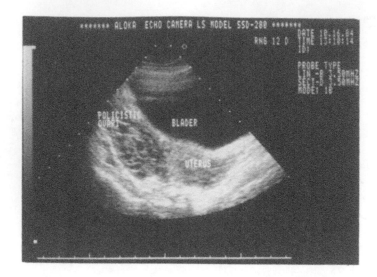

FIGURE 21.   Large polycystic ovary in a patient suffering from primary infertility. The ovary is filled with numerous small cycts and an increased stroma is also visible.

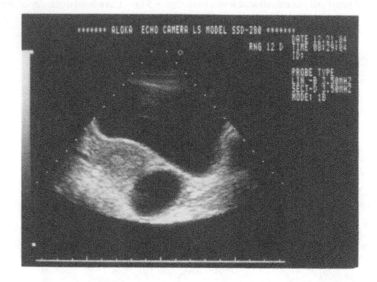

FIGURE 22.   A case of follicular cyst development. The daily growth rate was much higher than normal and the diameter of the follicle reached 32 mm on day 13 of the cycle.

ruptured follicle (LUF) syndrome is reported most extensively; the term was introduced in 1975 by Jewelewicz.[44] The main characteristic of this condition is complete luteinization of the follicle without ovulation and oocyte release. Etiology of LUF syndrome still remains unexplained. Actually, it seems that ovulation abnormality may be caused by either primary oocyte abnormality, abnormalities in prostaglandin synthesis, or defective midcycle LH surge.

Some evidence for primary oocyte abnormalities has been given by Liukkonen et al.,[45] who have attempted *in vitro* fertilization in three patients with proven persistent LUF syndrome. By performing follicular puncture they were able to collect only three ova from four treatment cycles. Of three preovulatory oocytes, two were morphologically abnormal, which made their fertilization impossible.

Clear evidence about the crucial role of prostaglandins for the rupture of preovulatory follicle also has been obtained. Parenteral application of an inhibitor of prostaglandin synthesis to estrus experimental animals always results in anovulation in spite of normal LH surge. The majority of unruptured follicles undergo luteinization, and it stands to reason that defective prostaglandin synthesis may play a role in the pathophysiology of LUF in otherwise normal menstrual cycles in humans.[27]

Recently, a group of American authors have reported a case of LUF syndrome with histological and hormonal documentation of the ovulation disorder in the rhesus monkey.[46] An interesting observation was the blunted midcycle LH surge and the absence of a normal progesterone increase in conjunction with gonadotrophin surge. Absence of the preovulatory progesterone increase seems to be a primary event, since it is known that a preovulatory rise of progesterone is required for the full expression of LH surge.[47] Pathophysiological examination of the unruptured follicle revealed complete luteinization. The oocyte within the follicle was immature and arrested in the first meiotic division.[46]

However, quoted experimental and clinical studies are either performed in a small number of cases or with experimental animals, and should not be directly extrapolated to clinical practice. Although these data are offering new insights into the pathophysiology of LUF syndrome, at the moment the etiology of this condition still remains obscure.

Frequency of LUF syndrome is, according to the reported data, extremely variable in potentially fertile women, and is estimated to be between 6 to 47%.[48,49] In endometriotic patients, the reported incidence of LUF was 11-33%.[50,51] In patients with infertility of unknown reason, the LUF syndrome was found in 60% of cases.[52] A particularly high incidence (up to 52%) was also reported in patients with chronic pelvic infection.[53] Obvious differences in estimated frequency of the condition can be partly attributed to the heterogenicity of investigated patients, different criteria for the normal ovulatory cycle, and non-uniform timing of laparoscopy.

LUF syndrome at first was diagnosed exclusively by laparoscopy. A pathognomonic laparoscopic finding was visualization of the follicular cyst with absent stigma in the luteal phase of the cycle. However, inappropriate timing of laparoscopy, later than 2 to 4 d after ovulation, may be an important cause of false-positive diagnosis of anovulation. At that time, the ovulatory stigma is easily covered by a new layer of cells, thus causing a failure in the diagnosis of ovulation.[54] Diagnostic accuracy of laparoscopy can be much improved by taking the sample of peritoneal fluid for biochemical analysis. A reliable sign of ovulation is the presence of follicular fluid which increases the levels of steroid hormones in the peritoneal fluid.[55]

Ultrasound diagnosis of LUF syndrome is based on daily observation of normal follicular development and normal diameter of the preovulatory follicle. During the period of expected ovulation, the follicle remains the same size or slightly larger, and maintains its tense appearance. Luteinization of the unruptured follicle is seen as progressive accumulation of strong echoes, predominately located in the periphery of the cyst (Figures 23 and 24).[56]

Although, ultrasound diagnosis of the LUF syndrome is considered to be relatively simple and accurate, the comparison of sonographic and laparoscopic findings provides some other facts.

Negative ultrasonic findings of LUF correlated well with laparoscopy without false negatives, but false-positive findings of the disease were found in 17% of cases.[45] This tendency of sonography to overestimate the frequency of the LUF syndrome may be explained by sonographic findings in normal ovulatory cycles. The ruptured follicle may be filled with fluid within several hours after ovulation without a significant decrease in its diameter. It may give the false impression of defective ovulation on repeated ultrasonic examination the

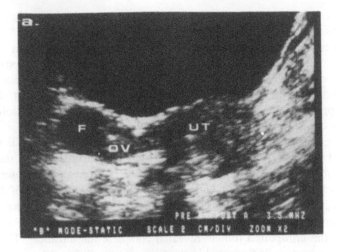

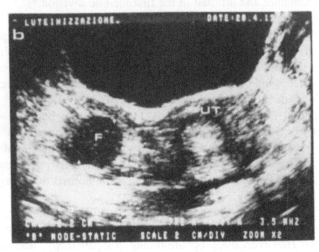

FIGURE 23.   Ultrasonic findings in a case of LUF syndrome. A mature ovarian follicle can be seen in the right ovary on day 14 of the cycle (a). The follicle is unruptured and slightly larger on day 15. The endometrium is echogenic and a small amount of fluid is present in the pouch of Douglas due to ovarian secretion (b). F, follicle; OV, ovary; UT, uterus. (Courtesy of Dr. D'Addario, Bari, Italy.)

following day.[30] Diagnostic error may also occur in the presence of an intraovarian cyst or hydrosalpinx. Such structures can be misinterpreted as an unruptured follicle, particularly if examinations are started later in the follicular phase on day 11 or 12.

V. ULTRASOUND EVALUATION OF STIMULATED CYCLES

Ovulation disorders are present in up to 25% of infertile patients. Inappropriate follicular maturation and anovulation are always the consequences of disruption in the precisely coordinated interaction between the components of the hypothalamic-pituitary-ovarian axis which have to operate within the strict quantitative limits and accurate temporal sequence of events throughout the menstrual cycle. The understanding of the basic mechanisms regulating the reproductive process prompted the development and use of effective drugs and hormones in modulating the function of the hypothalamic-pituitary-ovarian axis. The most

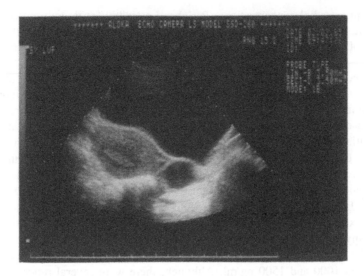

FIGURE 24. LUF syndrome. Note the presence of intrafollicular echoes within the apparently normal preovulatory follicle and increased endometrium echogenicity. The same finding persisted for a few days and diagnosis of LUF syndrome was made.

commonly used therapeutic agents in the field are clomiphene citrate, human menopausal gonadotropin (HMG), and gonadotropin-releasing hormone (Gn-RH). Each of these agents acts through different mechanisms, and optimal therapeutic effects can be achieved only after identification of the underlying cause of ovarian failure.

Clomiphene citrate modulates the hypothalamic-pituitary axis and increases endogenous FSH production, thus promoting the development of multiple mature preovulatory follicles. HMG exerts its action upon direct stimulation of the ovaries and promotes development of multiple follicles by overriding the mechanism of selection in the ovary.

Gonadotropin-releasing hormone or luteinizing hormone-releasing hormone stimulates the secretion of pituitary gonadotropins and is most effective for the treatment of hypothalamic amenorrhea.

The role of sonography in induced ovulation could be summarized as follows: detection of the number of developing follicles, assessment of the adequacy of follicular response and detection of ovulation, assistance of human chorionic gonadotropin administration timing, and detection of complications. The technique of ultrasound examinations is the same as in the spontaneous cycles. It is equally important to repeat examinations every day starting from the day 9 of the cycle, and all examinations should be performed by the same observer. The follicle growth rate in the stimulated cycle is similar to the spontaneous cycle, and the diameter of the dominant preovulatory follicle is insignificantly larger.[57,58] Detection of the number of developing follicles helps in the interpretation of peripheral plasma estradiol levels and may prevent the occurrence of multiple pregnancies when vast follicles are demonstrated.[59] However, there is poor correlation between the peripheral estradiol levels and the diameter of the dominant follicle in stimulated cycles.[60] It could easily be explained by the presence of multiple follicles, which contribute to overall estradiol production. Much better results were obtained when either the number of follicles larger than 10 mm or the total follicular volume was compared to the plasma estradiol.[61] An important limitation of these correlations is the variable responsiveness of the follicles to stimulation in terms of estrogen production capacity and distortion of follicular shape, due to mutual follicle compression. In spite of the described limitations, there is the common attitude that ultrasound is helpful for interpreting estradiol concentrations. Peripheral estradiol levels may reflect production of either single large preovulatory follicles or multiple immature follicles. With sonographic visualization of the ovaries this diagnostic probelm is effectively solved (Figure 25, Graph 4).

Furthermore, sonographic studies offer the advantage of easy orientation about therapy success, particularly in cases with poor follicular development. A typical finding in such cases is the demonstration of single or multiple follicles exhibiting slow or irregular growth pattern. Ultrasound also can provide data about insufficient ovulation regardless of the successful initiation of follicular growth and maturity. In both clomiphene and HMG-stimulated cycles, the defective ovulation is characterized by the presence of either luteinized or nonluteinized follicular cysts that fail to decrease in size after spontaneous LH surge or human chorionic gonadotropin (HCG) administration. [62,63] LUFs are resembling the ultrasonic appearance of LUF syndrome in the spontaneous cycles with the same diagnostic limitations as discussed extensively before (Figure 26).

HMG therapy requires the use of serial estradiol estimations and sonographic examinations to estimate the optimal time of HCG administration. Optimal estradiol concentrations are usually between 1000 and 1500 pg/ml. Although, there were several reports of successful HCG timing when the dominant follicle reached 18 mm or more in size, further experience indicated the follicle size alone cannot serve as a reliable parameter of follicular maturity. [64,65] It can be explained simply by the fact that the largest follicle does not always represent the most mature one in terms of estrogen synthesis and oocyte maturity. Optimal timing of HCG remains a particularly important part of ovulation induction because either premature or late application can be atretogenic and therefore can actively inhibit ovulation. [66] Because of this, simultaneous biochemical and biological assessments of follicle maturation are necessary for optimal results (Figure 27, Graphs 5 and 6).

The most important complication of ovulation induction is hyperstimulation. It is characterized by multiple follicles and development of luteal cysts after ovulation. Ovarian enlargement is always present in such cases and can be well documented by ultrasound. Sonographic measurement of the ovarian size is much superior to the clinical estimations, and enables better distinction between the patients who developed mild or moderate hyperstimulation. [67] However, mild to moderate hyperstimulation is regarded as an acceptable sequelae of ovulation induction, and does not cause significant complications except increased probability of multiple pregnancies (Figure 28).

On the contrary, severe hyperstimulation represents a potentially life-threatening condition. It is characterized by marked ovarian enlargement (over 10 cm in diameter) and presence of peritoneal and pleural effusions with symptoms of cardiovascular and renal failure. The development of severe ovarian hyperstimulation can be suspected in patients who develop numerous small follicles of similar size as early as days 8 and 9 of the cycle. Clear evidence of continuous ovarian enlargement over the next few days indicates a high risk of ovarian hyperstimulation syndrome development. [68] If such a finding is accompanied by high estradiol levels above 2000 pg/ml, an HCG injection should be withheld to avoid full expression of symptoms (Figures 29 and 30).

VI. CONCLUSION

Ultrasound monitoring of follicular growth and ovulation has become an important method in the management of female infertility. Potential benefits of the use of sonography in the assessment of spontaneous and induced cycles have been well documented during the last several years. A new technical achievement, the transvaginal probe, will probably contribute to further expansion of ultrasound diagnostics in this field. The use of the transvaginal probe alleviates the need for the full bladder technique and provides a high-resolution image of

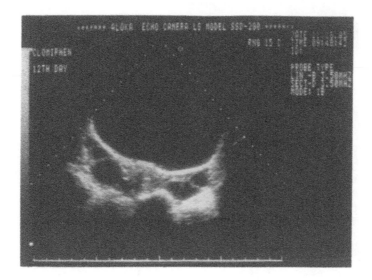

A

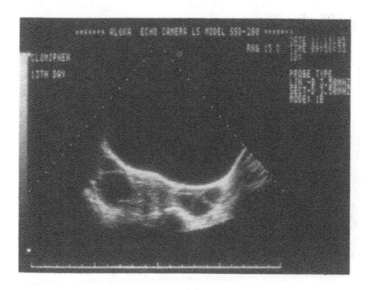

B

FIGURE 25. Transverse sonogram performed on day 12 of the cycle in a patient receiving clomiphene stimulation. The right ovary contains the dominant follicle and three more follicles are seen in the left ovary. (A) The same patient on day 13. The mean diameter of the dominant follicle reached 22 mm and the other four follicles also increased. (B) On the following day, only one follicle was observed in the right ovary. The other four follicles disappeared completely. Normal ovulation has taken place. (C) One day later, one can observe the reappearance of cystic structures representing the corpora lutea in the ovaries. (D) This clearly illustrates the importance of daily examinations for successful diagnosis of ovulation.

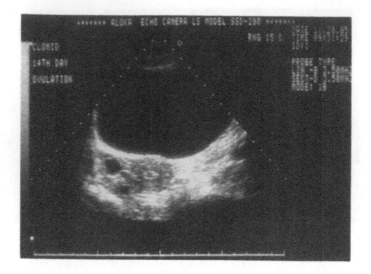

FIGURE 25C.

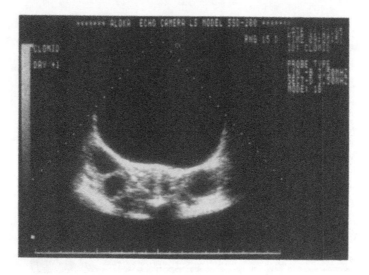

FIGURE 25D.

the ovaries. This makes examinations more simple and convenient than before. Moreover, ultrasound examination thus becomes a logical extension of clinical examination, and this will, without doubt, result in better understanding of ovarian physiology and further refinement of therapeutic approaches.

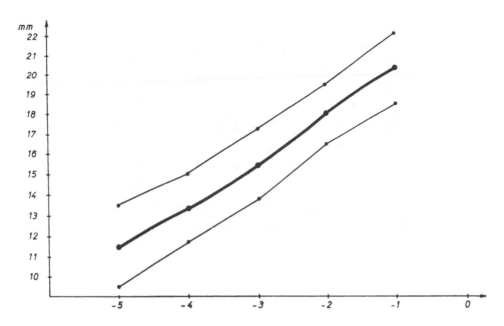

GRAPH 4. The diameter of the largest follicle (mean ± SD) in clomiphene-stimulated cycles from days −5 to −1. Day 0 = ovulation; N = 20.

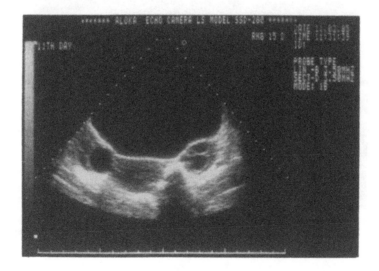

A

FIGURE 26. A case of unsuccessful ovulation induction with clomiphene. On day 11 of the cycle, sonographic examination demonstrated satisfactory response to the therapy. Three developing follicles were present within the ovaries. (A) On day 14 of the cycle, the follicles reached 25 to 30 mm in size (B), but ovulation has not taken place on the following day, and the follicles remained of the same size and maintained their tense appearance (C).

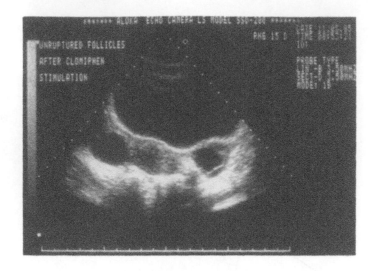

FIGURE 26B.

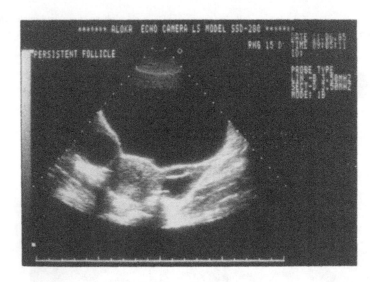

FIGURE 26C.

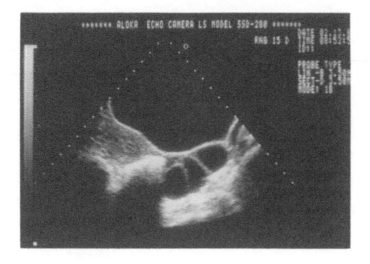

A

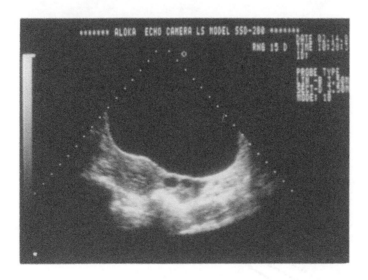

B

FIGURE 27. Successful induction of ovulation with HMG + HCG therapy. Three large preovulatory follicles are visible in the left ovary (A) and almost completely disappeared on the next day (B).

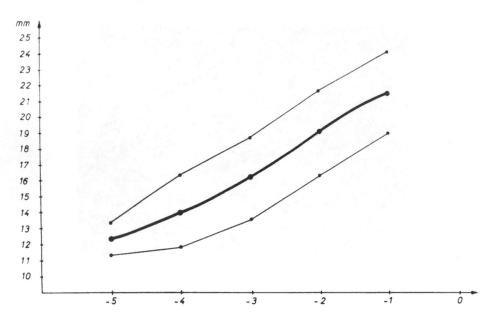

GRAPH 5. The diameter of the largest follicle (mean ± SD) in HMG + HCG-stimulated cycles. Day 0 = ovulation; N = 20.

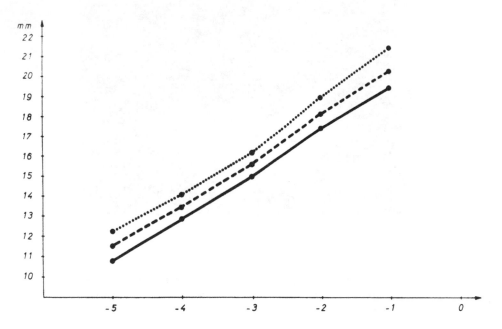

GRAPH 6. Mean follicular diameter in spontaneous and stimulated cycles from days −5 to −1 as related to the day of ovulation.

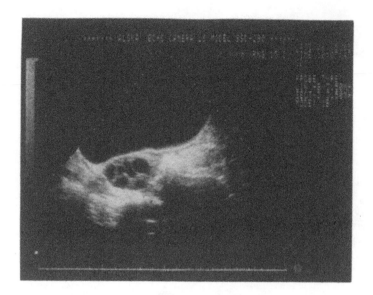

FIGURE 28. Oblique scan showing the enlarged ovary filled with numerous follicles in a case of moderate hyperstimulation after HMG therapy.

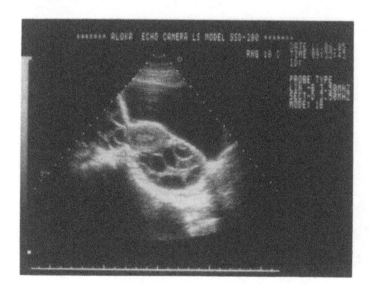

A

FIGURE 29. A case of severe ovarian hyperstimulation after HMG and HCG ovulation induction. Transverse scan of the patient 2 d after HCG administration shows bilateral ovarian enlargement and vast follicles present within them. (A) Further increase in the size of the left ovary is demonstrated on longitudinal scan performed on the following day. (B) After 10 d, the ovaries were 15 to 20 cm in average size and large luteal cysts were clearly visible (C).

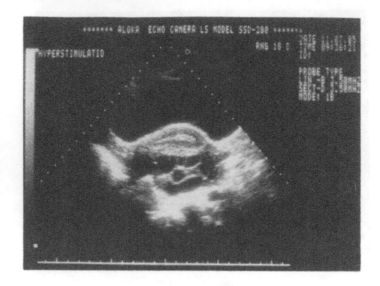

FIGURE 29B.

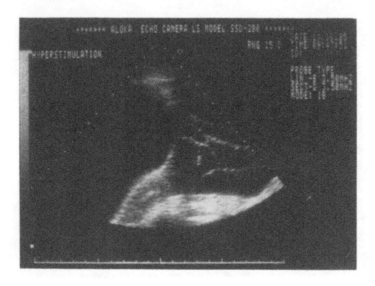

FIGURE 29C.

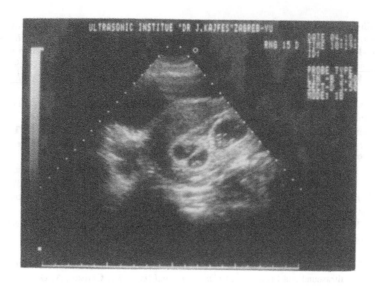

FIGURE 30. Triplet pregnancy in an infertile patient after induction of ovulation with HMG.

REFERENCES

1. **Kratochwil, A., Urban, G., and Friedrich, G.,** Ultrasonic tomography of the ovary, *Ann. Chir. Gynaecol. Fenn.,* 61, 211, 1972.
2. **Hackelöer, B. J., Nitschke-Debelstein, S., Daume, E., Sturm, G., and Bucholz, R.,** Ultraschalldarstellung von Ovarderänderungen bei Gonadotropin Stimulierung, *Geburtshilfe Frauenheilkd.,* 37, 185, 1977.
3. **Fleischer, A. C., Darnell, J., Rodier, J., Lindsay, A., and James, A. E.,** Sonographic monitoring of ovarian follicular development, *J. Clin. Ultrasound,* 9, 275, 1981.
4. **O'Herlihy, C., de Crespigny, L., and Robinson, H. P.,** Monitoring ovarian follicular development with real-time ultrasound, *Br. J. Obstet. Gynaecol.,* 87, 613, 1980.
5. **Queenan, J. T., O'Brien, G. D., Bains, L. M., Simpson, J., Collins, W. P., and Campbell, S.,** Ultrasound scanning of ovaries to detect ovulation in women, *Fertil. Steril.,* 34, 99, 1980.
6. **Goswamy, R. K., Campbell, S., and Whitehead, M. I.,** Screening for ovarian cancer, *Clin. Obstet. Gynecol.,* 10, 621, 1983.
7. **Hackelöer, B. J. and Nitschke-Debelstein, S.,** Ovarian imaging by ultrasound: an attempt to define a reference plane, *J. Clin. Ultrasound,* 8, 497, 1980.
8. **Christie, A. D.,** *Ultrasound and Infertility,* Chartwel-Bratt, Bromley, 1981, 19.
9. **Hillier, S. G., Reichert, L. E., and Van, E. V.,** Control of preovulatory follicular estrogen biosynthesis in the human ovary, *J. Clin. Endocrinol. Metab.,* 52, 847, 1981.
10. **Hsueh, A. J. W., Jones, P. B. C., Adashi, E. Y., Wang, C., Zhuang, Z., and Welsh, T. H.,** Intraovarian mechanisms in the hormonal control of granulosa cell differentiation in rats, *J. Reprod. Fertil.,* 69, 325, 1983.
11. **Geisthövel, F., Klosa, W., Rabold, B., Schillinger, H., and Breckwoldt, M.,** Further sonographical and endocrine aspects of physiological and insufficient ovarian function, in *Recent Advances in Ultrasound Diagnosis,* Vol. 4, Kurjak, A. and Kossoff, G., Eds., Excerpta Medica, Amsterdam, 1984, 230.
12. **Di Zerega, G. S., Turner, C. K., Stouffer, R. L., Anderson, L. D., Channing, C. P., and Hodgen, G. D.,** Suppression of follicle-stimulating hormone-dependent folliculogenesis during the primate ovarian cycle, *J. Clin. Endocrinol. Metab.,* 52, 451, 1981.
13. **Ross, G. T. and Schreiber, J. R.,** The ovary, in *Reproductive Endocrinology,* Yen, S. S. C. and Jaffe, R. B., Eds., W.B. Saunders, Philadelphia, 1986, 115.

14. **O'Herlihy, C., de Crespigny, L., Lopata, A., Johnston, I., Hoult, I., and Robinson, H.,** Preovulatory follicular size: a comparison of ultrasound and laparoscopic measurements, *Fertil. Steril.*, 34, 24, 1980.

15. **Funduk-Kurjak, B. and Kurjak, A.,** Ultrasound monitoring of follicular maturation and ovulation in normal menstrual cycles and ovulation induction, *Acta Obstet. Gynecol. Scand.*, 61, 329, 1982.

16. **Ritchie, W. G. M.,** Ultrasound in the evaluation of normal and induced ovulation, *Fertil. Steril.*, 43, 167, 1985.

17. **Baird, D. T. and Fraser, I. S.,** Blood production and ovarian secretion rate of estradiol and estrone in women throughout the menstrual cycle, *J. Clin. Endocrinol. Metab.*, 38, 1009, 1974.

18. **Hackelöer, B. J., Fleming, R., Robinson, H. P., Adam, A. H., and Coutts, J. R. T.,** Correlation of ultrasonic and endocrinologic parameters of human follicular development, *Am. J. Obstet. Gynecol.*, 135, 122, 1979.

19. **Buttery, B., Trounson, A., McMaster, R., and Wood, C.,** Evaluation of diagnostic ultrasound as a parameter of follicular development in an in vitro fertilization program, *Fertil. Steril.*, 39, 458, 1983.

20. **Hoff, J. D., Lasley, B. L., Wang, C. F., and Yen, S. S. C.,** The two pools of pituitary gonadotropin: regulation during the menstrual cycle, *J. Clin. Endocrinol. Metab.*, 44, 302, 1977.

21. **Yen, S. S. C. and Lein, A.,** The apparent paradox of the negative and positive feedback control of gonadotropin secretion, *Am. J. Obstet. Gynecol.*, 126, 942, 1976.

22. **Blandau, R. J.,** Anatomy of ovulation, *Clin. Obstet. Gynecol.*, 10, 347, 1969.

23. **Bomsel-Helmreich, O., Bessis, R., Vu, N., and Huyen, L.,** Cumulus oophorus of the preovulatory follicle assessed by ultrasound and histology, in *Ultrasound and Infertility,* Christie, A. D., Ed., Chartwel-Bratt, Bromley, 1981, 105.

24. **Kerin, J. F., Edmonds, D. K., Warnes, G. M., Cox, L. W., Seamark, R. F., Matthews, C. D., Young, G. B., and Baird, D. T.,** Morphological and functional relationships of graafian follicle growth to ovulation in women using ultrasonic, laparoscopic and biochemical measurements, *Br. J. Obstet. Gynaecol.*, 88, 81, 1981.

25. **Lenz, S.,** Ultrasonic study of follicular maturation, ovulation and development of corpus luteum during normal menstrual cycles, *Acta Obstet. Gynecol. Scand.*, 64, 15, 1985.

26. **Picker, R. H., Smith, D. H., Tucker, M. H., and Saunder, D. M.,** Ultrasonic signs of imminent ovulation, *J. Clin. Ultrasound*, 11, 1, 1983.

27. **Bomsel-Helmreich, O. and Huyen, L. V. N.,** Delayed ovulation without inhibition of LH surge in the rabbit: a model of atresia of the preovulatory follicle, in *Follicular Maturation and Ovulation,* Rolland, R., van Hall, E. V., Hillier, S. G., McNatty, K. P., and Schoemaker, J., Eds., Excerpta Medica, Amsterdam, 1982, 295.

28. **Doyle, J. B.,** Exploratory culdotomy for observation of tubo-ovarian physiology at ovulation, *Fertil. Steril.*, 2, 475, 1951.

29. **Espey, L. L. and Lipner, H.,** Measurements of intrafollicular pressure in the rabbit ovary, *Am. J. Physiol.*, 205, 1067, 1963.

30. **De Crespigny, L., O'Herlihy, C., and Robinson, H. P.,** Ultrasonic observation of the mechanism of human ovulation, *Am. J. Obstet. Gynecol.*, 139, 177, 1981.

31. **Sakamoto, C. and Nakano, H.,** The echogenic endometrium and alterations during the menstrual cycle, *Int. J. Gynecol. Obstet.*, 20, 255, 1982.

32. **Hackelöer, B. J.,** The role of ultrasound in female infertility management, *Ultrasound Med. Biol.*, 10, 35, 1984.

33. **Fleischer, A. C., Kalameris, C. C., and Entman, S. S.,** Sonographic depiction of the endometrium during normal cycles, in *Proceedings of the Fourth Meeting of the World Federation for Ultrasound in Medicine and Biology,* Gill, R. W. and Dadd, M. J., Eds., Pergamon Press, Sydney, 1985, 281.

34. **Zander, J. and Ober, G. K.,** Presence of glycogen in the endometria of castrated women following administration of progesterone, *Arch. Gynaekol.*, 196, 481, 1962.

35. **Crade, M., Patel, J., and McQuown, D.,** Sonographic imaging of the glycogen stage of fetal choroid plexus, *Am. J. Radiol.*, 137, 489, 1981.

36. **Fleischer, A. C., Muhletaler, C., and James, A. E.,** Sonographic patterns in normal and abnormal bowel, *RCNA,* 18, 145, 1980.

37. **Swanson, M., Sauerbrei, E. E., and Cooperberg, P. L.,** Medical implications of ultrasonically detected polycystic ovaries, *J. Clin. Ultrasound*, 9, 219, 1981.

38. **Parisi, L., Tramonti, M., and Casciano, S.,** The role of ultrasound in the study of polycystic ovarian disease, *J. Clin. Ultrasound*, 10, 167, 1982.

39. **Hann, L. E., Hall, D. A., McArdle, C. R., and Seibel, M.,** Polycystic ovarian disease: sonographic spectrum, *Radiology,* 150, 531, 1984.

40. **Tabbakh, G. H., Lofty, I., and Azab, I.,** Correlation of the ultrasonic appearance of the ovaries in polycystic ovarian disease and the clinical, hormonal and laparoscopic findings, *Am. J. Obstet. Gynecol.*, 154, 892, 1986.

41. **Franks, S., Adams, J., Mason, H., and Polson, D.,** Ovulatory disorders in women with polycystic ovary syndrome, *Clin. Obstet. Gynecol.,* 12, 605, 1985.
42. **Polan, M. L., Totora, M., Caldwell, B. V., deCherney, A. H., Haseltine, F. P., and Kase, N.,** Abnormal ovarian cycles as diagnosed by ultrasound and serum estradiol levels, *Fertil. Steril.,* 37, 342, 1982.
43. **Coutts, J. R. T., Adam, A. H., and Fleming, R.,** Ovarian ultrasound and endocrine profiles in women with unexplained infertility, in *Ultrasound and Infertility,* Christie, A. D., Ed., Chartwell-Bratt, Bromley, 1981, 89.
44. **Jewelewicz, R.,** Management of infertility resulting from anovulation, *Am. J. Obstet. Gynecol.,* 122, 309, 1975.
45. **Liukkonen, S., Koskimies, A. I., Tenhunen, A., and Ylostalo, P.,** Luteinized unruptured follicle (LUF) syndrome, *J. Fr. Echogr.,* 3, 285, 1986.
46. **Schenken, R. S., Werlin, L. B., Williams, R. F., Prihoda, T. J., and Hodgen, G. D.,** Histologic and hormonal documentation of the luteinized unruptured follicle syndrome, *Am. J. Obstet. Gynecol.,* 154, 839, 1986.
47. **Liu, J. H. and Yen, S. S. C.,** Induction of midcycle gonadotropin surge by ovarian steroid in women: a critical reevaluation, *J. Clin. Endocrinol. Metab.,* 57, 907, 1983.
48. **Kerin, J. F., Kirby, C., Morris, D., McEvoy, M., Ward, B., and Cox, L. W.,** Incidence of luteinized unruptured follicle phenomenon in cycling women, *Fertil. Steril.,* 40, 620, 1983.
49. **Varnell, J. A., Balasch, J., Fuster, J. S., and Fuster, R.,** Ovulation in fertile women, *Fertil. Steril.,* 37, 712, 1982.
50. **Thomas, E. J., Lenton, E. A., and Cooke, I. D.,** Follicle growth patterns and endocrinological abnormalities in infertile women with minor degrees of endometriosis, *Br. J. Obstet. Gynaecol.,* 93, 852, 1986.
51. **Brosens, I. A., Koninckx, P. R., and Corvelyn, P. A.,** A study of plasma progesterone, estradiol, prolactin and LH levels and luteal appearance of the ovaries in patients with endometriosis and infertility, *Br. J. Obstet. Gynaecol.,* 85, 246, 1978.
52. **Koninckx, P. R., Heyens, W. J., Corvelyn, P. A., and Brosens, I. A.,** Delayed onset of luteinization as a cause of infertility, *Fertil. Steril.,* 29, 266, 1978.
53. **Hamilton, C. J. C. M., Evers, J. L. H., and Hoogland, H. J.,** Ovulatory disorders and inflammatory adnexal damage: a neglected cause of the failure of fertility microsurgery, *Br. J. Obstet. Gynaecol.,* 93, 282, 1986.
54. **Portuondo, J. A., Augustin, A., Herran, C., and Echanojauregui, A. D.,** The corpus luteum in infertile patients found during laparoscopy, *Fertil. Steril.,* 36, 37, 1981.
55. **Traina, V., Miniello, G., D'Addario, V., and Kurjak, A.,** New approaches in the diagnosis of the LUF syndrome, in *Recent Advances in Ultrasound Diagnosis,* Vol. 4, Kurjak, A. and Kossoff, G., Eds., Excerpta Medica, Amsterdam, 1984, 264.
56. **Coulam, C. B., Hill, L. M., and Breckle, R.,** Ultrasonic evidence for luteinization of unruptured preovulatory follicle, *Fertil. Steril.,* 37, 524, 1982.
57. **O'Herlihy, C., Pepperell, R. J., and Robinson, H. P.,** Ultrasound timing of human chorionic gonadotropin administration in clomiphene stimulated cycles, *Obstet. Gynecol.,* 59, 40, 1982.
58. **Marrs, R. P., Vargyas, J. M., and March, C. M.,** Ultrasonic and endocrinologic measurements in hMG therapy, *Am. J. Obstet. Gynecol.,* 145, 417, 1983.
59. **Muse, K. and Wilson, E. A.,** Monitoring ovulation induction: use of biochemical and biophysical parameters, *Semin. Reprod. Endocrinol.,* 4, 301, 1986.
60. **Haning, R. V., Austin, C. W., Kuzma, D. L., Shapiro, S. S., and Zweibel, W. J.,** Ultrasound evaluation of estrogen monitoring for induction of ovulation with menotropins, *Fertil. Steril.,* 37, 627, 1982.
61. **Mantzavinos, T., Garcia, J. E., and Jones, H. W.,** Ultrasound measurement of ovarian follicles stimulated by human gonadotropins for oocyte recovery and in vitro fertilization, *Fertil. Steril.,* 40, 461, 1983.
62. **Coulam, C. B., Hill, L. M., and Breckle, R.,** Ultrasonic assessment of subsequent unexplained infertility after ovulation induction, *Br. J. Obstet. Gynaecol.,* 90, 460, 1983.
63. **Stanger, J. D. and Yovich, J. L.,** Failure of human oocyte release at ovulation, *Fertil. Steril.,* 41, 827, 1984.
64. **Sundström, P., Persson, P. H., Liedholm, P., and Wramsby, H.,** The ability of ultrasound to determine the time for harvesting preovulatory oocytes, *Acta Obstet. Gynecol. Scand.,* 62, 219, 1983.
65. **Messinis, I. E. and Templeton, A.,** Urinary estrogen levels and follicle ultrasound measurements in clomiphene induced cycles with an endogenous luteinizing hormone surge, *Br. J. Obstet. Gynaecol.,* 93, 43, 1986.
66. **Williams, R. F. and Hodgen, G. D.,** Disparate effects of human chorionic gonadotropin during the late follicular phase in monkeys: normal ovulation, follicular atresia, ovarian acyclicity and hypersecretion of follicle-stimulating hormone, *Fertil. Steril.,* 33, 64, 1980.
67. **McArdle, C., Siebel, M., Hann, L., Weinstein, F., and Taymor, M.,** The diagnosis of ovarian hyperstimulation (OHS): the impact of ultrasound, *Fertil. Steril.,* 39, 464, 1983.

68. **Rankin, R. N. and Hutton, L. C.,** Ultrasound in the ovarian hyperstimulation syndrome, *J. Clin. Ultrasound,* 9, 473, 1981.
69. **Renaud, R. L., Maclere, J., and Dervain, I.,** Echographic study of follicular maturation and ovulation during the normal menstrual cycle, *Fertil. Steril.,* 33, 272, 1980.
70. **Ylostalo, P., Ronnenberg, L., and Jouppila, P.,** Measurement of ovarian follicle by ultrasound in ovulation induction, *Fertil. Steril.,* 31, 61, 1979.
71. **Hall, D. A., Hann, L. E., Ferruci, J. T., and Black, E. B.,** Sonographic morphology of the normal menstrual cycle, *Radiology,* 133, 185, 1979.

Chapter 5

TRANSVAGINAL SONOGRAPHY IN THE MANAGEMENT OF INFERTILITY

Ilan E. Timor-Tritsch and Shraga Rottem

TABLE OF CONTENTS

I. INTRODUCTION

Infertility is a major disorder affecting approximately one in six couples. One in six infertile women have mechanical infertility, half of whom are affected by inadequate ovulatory function.

The large number of affected couples has led to increased research into the causes and treatments. One of the most valuable tools in diagnosis and treatment is ultrasound. The first ultrasound-guided oocyte retrieval was reported by Lenz et al.[1] Ultrasound-aided follicular size determination was first correlated to serum estradiol concentrations by Hackelöer et al.[2] Several years later in 1984, Dellenbach et al.[3] introduced oocyte retrieval by means of a transvaginal probe.

In this chapter, a brief overview of the pertinent physics will be attempted to describe the clinical use of the transvaginal probe in general and in the diagnostic as well as the invasive management of the infertile patient in particular. The general technique of transvaginal sonography (TVS) is then described. Scanning of the uterus, the fallopian tubes, and the ovaries is followed by a brief description of follicular maturation (natural or hormonally induced) monitoring by the means of TVS. Finally, the TVS-guided oocyte retrieval for *in vitro* fertilization (IVF) and embryo transfer (ET) will be presented.

II. PHYSICAL CONSIDERATIONS

Frequency is one of the most important variables to consider in the production of a high-resolution image. It is directly related to the axial and lateral resolution. (The two-point discrimination capability of the transducer becomes better with increased frequencies.) However, if the frequency is raised, the tissue attenuation is higher; hence, deeper structures will be progressively less defined.

Focal range is the region where the picture is displayed at its best on the screen. Focal distance is the span from the tip of the transducer to the point where the clearest image is created. Both are inversely related to frequency. The focal range of a typical 3.5-MHz probe, therefore, is about 7 to 18 cm with a focal distance of about 12 cm, making it ideal for transabdominal scanning. A 6.5-MHz probe, on the other hand, has a focal range of 2 to 7 cm with the acoustic focus at 4 to 5 cm. Image clarity is determined by the axial (linear) and lateral (azimutal) resolutions. Image quality, resolution, and transducer frequency are directly related to each other. The lateral resolution of a 3.5-MHz probe is close to 2 mm, the axial resolution being 0.6 mm. The appropriate values for the 6.5-MHz probe are 1.3 and 0.5 mm (or better), respectively. By requirements of physical law, imaging of deeper pelvic structures through the abdominal route is best achieved with the use of a 3.5- or at most a 5.0-MHz probe. The inherent reduction of focal depth and increased attenuation would limit the use of a transabdominally applied higher frequency transducer even though image quality should potentially improve.

The transvaginal route allows the use of a higher frequency by applying the probe directly into the vaginal vault, close to the pelvic organs. In this way, one takes advantage of the closer focal range (2 to 4 cm) of this transducer crystal, enhancing picture resolution and clinical efficiency. Most of the work presented here was performed with a 6.5- (Elscint, Ltd., Haifa, Israel) and a 5.0-MHz (General Electric, U.S.) transvaginal transducer probe.

III. HOW TVS IS PERFORMED

The first step is giving the patient adequate information about the examination. Then, the probe is lubricated with coupling gel and inserted into a protective rubber sheet (e.g., a condom or a surgical glove, using one of its digits). A second layer of coupling material is

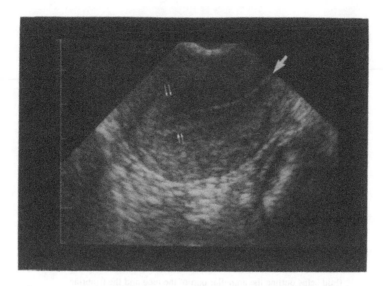

FIGURE 1. Longitudinal section of a normal uterus: the cervix is on the right upper side of the picture. Note the uniform echogenicity of the myometrium and the regular cavity line (arrow). The endometrium (small double arrows) measures 9 mm.

then applied to the tip of the probe, which is then inserted into the vagina. A word of caution: the group headed by Schwimmer[4] have reported that there are spermicidal properties associated with the commonly used commercial sonic coupling gels. Therefore, the use of a saline solution is advised for lubrication and coupling.

The controls of the machine and the recording equipment are then set to save on the actual examination time. The patient should be placed in a slightly reversed Trendelenburg position to facilitate the pooling into the pelvis of the normally present (or other) intra-abdominal fluid. This can help in creating fluid/organ interfaces to better outline the target organs. A more detailed presentation of the scanning technique was presented elsewhere in the literature.[5] However, one of the maneuvers aiding the diagnosis should be mentioned here. If the tip of the probe is pointed toward a pelvic organ or pelvic mass and pressure is exerted upon it, this structure moves up in the pelvis. If the pressure is then released, the organ or mass slides back to its original site. This sliding movement is evident if one relates this to another, relatively stationary structure or the pelvic floor. We refer to this dynamic finding, which may be used to diagnose adhesions in the pelvis, as the "sliding organs sign".[5]

IV. SCANNING THE REPRODUCTIVE ORGANS

A. The Uterus

Determinations of position and size can be somewhat better performed by transabdominal sonography. However, examinations of the myometrium, endometrial lining, uterine contents, and structure for noting the presence of malformation should be done via the transvaginal route (Figure 1). Endometrial grading or the diagnosis of a relatively small (1 cm) intramural or submucous fibroid is an easy task for TVS. Blood clots, intracavitary fluid collection, or retained products of concept also may be diagnosed. Endometrial polyps or any irregularity of the discrete "cavity-line" may be observed.

B. The Fallopian Tube

If healthy and normal without surrounding fluid, the fallopian tube cannot be seen with the equipment presently available. In the presence of pelvic fluid, chances are that it can

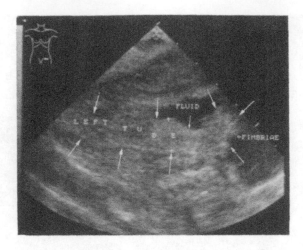

FIGURE 2.   The left tube is imaged. A small amount of pelvic
fluid helps outline the ampullar part of the tube and the fimbriae.

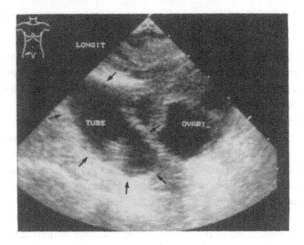

FIGURE 3.   TVS picture of hydrosalpinx. Note the dilated fluid-
filled right tube adjacent to a large hormonally stimulated follicle.

be visualized as an approximately 1-cm tortuous structure (Figure 2). Usually only parts of
it at a time are imaged due to this tortuosity. If not filled with fluid or a gestational sac,
the lumen cannot be seen. Any kind of intraluminal fluid (i.e., blood, serous, or purulent
material) facilitates the diagnosis of hemato-, pyo-, or hydrosalpinx (Figure 3).[6]

Acute inflammatory processes of the tube, alone or in combination with the ovary, present
a typical picture of a "conglomerate", including the dilated and fluid-filled tube "embrac-
ing" the ovary (Figure 4). Later in the evolution of this inflammatory process, the tubo-
ovarian abscess appears as a multilocular cystic structure in which the tube and the ovary
are beyond recognition. Motion tenderness can be elicited by pushing the probe under direct
and continuous observation toward the pelvic mass in question. This may help in the differential diagnosis of this disease.

The early and reliable diagnosis of tubal gestation is not only possible, but constitutes
one of the major strengths of TVS (Figure 5). Its detailed description is beyond the scope
of this chapter, but has been presented elsewhere.[7]

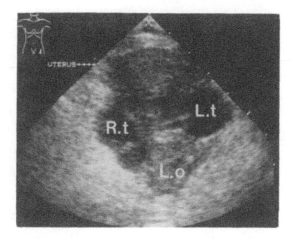

FIGURE 4. Typical picture of a bilaterial tubo-ovarian inflammatory process. The dilated and fluid-filled right and left tubes (R.t and L.t) as well as the left ovary (L.o) are shown behind the uterus.

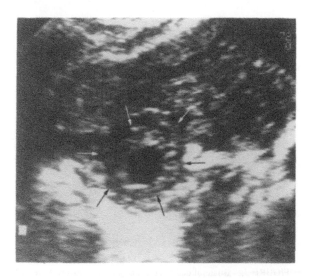

FIGURE 5. Left tubal pregnancy at $6^1/_2$ weeks. The thickened tubal wall is marked by small arrows. The sonolucent gestational sac is clearly visible.

C. The Ovary

Its relatively well-defined surface and steady shape, as well as its "sonographic marker", the follicles, renders the ovary an easy target for TVS (Figure 6). A detailed description of ovarian masses does not serve the purpose of this presentation; therefore, the interested reader is referred to the pertinent literature.[8,9] However, one should remember that in many instances the reason for the infertility may be ovarian pathology such as a cyst or a chronic inflammatory process with adhesive sequelae. These adhesions may be detected with the previously described "sliding organs sign".

Three entities should be mentioned here because of their relative significance: the corpus luteum, the polycystic ovary, and the endometroid cyst.

The corpus luteum can be described as being almost spheric, usually measuring 2 to 3

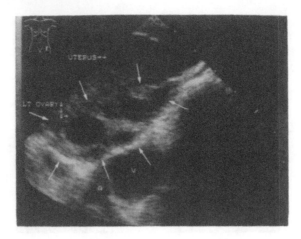

FIGURE 6.   The normal-size left ovary (small arrows) is out-lined below the uterus. Its sonographic markers, the Graffian follicles, make it easy to be localized during the reproductive years. The cross-section of the left hypogastric vein (V) and artery (A) are also seen.

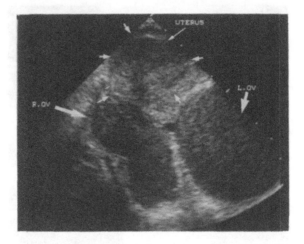

FIGURE 7.   Bilateral endometroid cysts (large arrows) are vis-ualized behind the uterus (small arrows). The uniform echogen-icity of these cysts is typical and due to the presence of blood.

cm, and conceivably reaching a diameter of 4 to 6 cm. If its diameter does not exceed 2 to 3 cm, its wall may show various degrees of thickening. Ovarian tissue (marked by the presence of follicles) should be looked for to differentiate it from other pathologies. The diversity of the contents of the corpus luteum is truly amazing: it may appear as trabecular, spike-like, nodular, and last but not least, completely sonolucent. The main differential diagnostic problem arises when one is asked to decide whether this structure is a "tubal ring" (i.e., tubal pregnancy) or a recent corpus luteum.

The sonographic image of polycystic ovaries is typical and seems to be pathognomonic. Large numbers of small (3 to 6 mm) follicles are "crowded" standing out at the surface of the enlarged ovaries.

The endometroid cyst (Figure 7) should be touched upon since it has a direct significance as one of the major causes of infertility. In spite of the fact that the structural appearance

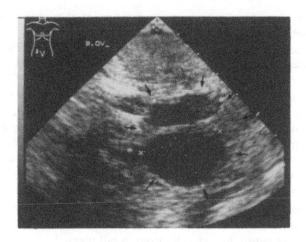

FIGURE 8. A dominant and a smaller follicle are shown within the right ovary on day 14 of a natural cycle.

of the dermoid and the endometroid cysts is similar (i.e., spheric, moderately and homogeneously echogenic), the diagnosis can be made by using the clinical information.

V. MONITORING OF FOLLICULAR MATURATION AND OVULATION INDUCTION

Due to the ability of ultrasonography to determine the exact timing of follicular maturation, it is an essential tool in the decision-making process when following, managing, and inducing ovulation. Its benefit lies in the fact that it is a relatively simple, accurate, and noninvasive measurement. Follicular size should be about 10 mm in average diameter in order to be visualized by the customary 3.5-MHz transabdominal probe. This occurs at or shortly after day 6 of a natural or induced cycle.

A normal dominant follicle grows at a rate of about 2 mm/day, reaching an average of 20 mm in diameter (range 18 to 24 mm) shortly before ovulation occurs.[10] In hormonally induced cycles, the total follicular volume shows the highest correlation with serum estradiol, since the rate of growth of the dominant follicle (Figure 8) or the other individual follicles is subject to changes during the cycle.[10] Timing of the ovulation induction agent (human chorionic gonadotropin HCG) injection is critical, since if administered prematurely, i.e., at a follicular size of 13 mm or less, the result is premature atresia of the follicle and hence, a shortened luteal phase.

Most centers perform daily scanning in order to follow the maturational changes of the follicles. Some centers also grade the endometrium along the cycle as an additional monitoring tool.[11]

Increasingly, TVS is being used to follow these follicular changes across the cycle. The sole determining factor in whether TVS is used over transabdominal sonography (TAS) seems to be the availability of transvaginal probes. The procedure is simple, easy to master, and presents "logistical" advantages to a busy ultrasound or IVF/ET unit, such as eliminating the need to wait for a full bladder.

Two potential procedural pitfalls have to be mentioned here. First, it is difficult to locate the ovaries quickly. They usually are found in the space between the posterolateral wall of the uterus and the easily located "large" hypogastric vein and artery (Figure 6). Therefore, it is advisable to start the scanning by first locating one of these structures. It also should be remembered that following previous pelvic surgery, the ovaries may be found in different and slightly unusual sites. Also, in a fraction of the cases they may only be found by employing the transabdominal scanning route.

The second is the problem of distinguishing ovarian anatomy. A few anatomical structures may assume the looks of an ovarian follicle. These include the cross section of the large pelvic vessels, the bowel, a possible hydrosalpinx, and an ovary with a cyst. The blood vessels can be recognized by their pulsatility and rotation of the probe by 90°; this provides a longitudinal section of the vessel which will prove its nature. The bowel, if observed for some time, will show peristalsis. The hydrosalpinx and the ovarian cysts are harder to differentiate from a follicle, but serial measurements usually help since these structures do not grow over time in the menstrual cycle. With careful consideration and a minimal amount of experience with TVS, these should not present serious problems to the sonographer.

TVS can easily detect minute amounts of pelvic fluid; therefore, the sudden appearance of previously nonexistent fluid in the cul-de-sac is indirect proof of recent ovulation. One must remember, though, that small amounts of pelvic fluid can be seen in the pouch of Douglas throughout, but mostly in midcycle, even in pill users.[12]

VI. TVS-GUIDED OOCYTE RETRIEVAL

There is an increasing popularity in the use of the transvaginal probe and the transvaginal route for egg retrieval in the IVF and ET programs throughout the entire world. The main reasons for this are reduced cost since it can be done on an outpatient basis; avoidance of general anesthesia with its attendant risks; and eliminating laparoscopy, which is potentially more dangerous.

The transvaginal approach for oocyte retrieval was introduced by Dellenbach et al.[3] in 1984. In their latest report, Feichtinger and Kemeter[16] reported on a 98.3% retrival rate in 61 patients using TVS. In this group, an average of 4.5 oocytes were aspirated per patient in contrast to 3.6 ova per patient in 371 women using TAS.

The authors' experience with a group of 127 patients at the Rambam Medical Center, Haifa, Israel, was similar.

The procedure itself is simple. After the patient has emptied her bladder, she is placed on a treatment table in lithotomy position. The vagina is cleaned, and the pelvis is covered with sterile drapes. After covering the vaginal transducer with a sterile glove, as described before, it is inserted in the vagina for an initial scan (Figure 9). On the screen, the software-generated biopsy line is aligned with the target follicles (Figure 10A). The follicle is then entered with the appropriate needle (Figure 10B) and the aspiration performed. The needle placement, the shrinking of the follicle during the process of aspiration, as well as the flushing of the follicle are clearly pictured (Figure 10C).

We attribute several important advantages to the transvaginal over the transabdominal follicular aspiration method:

1. The distance to the ovary is shorter
2. Higher-resolution pictures of the ovary and the follicles are produced
3. There is a smaller chance to injure the bowel and the blood vessels since the needle travels a shorter distance
4. The procedure is less painful
5. The bladder is not entered
6. No general anesthesia is needed
7. The procedure is significantly shorter
8. The cost is projected to be lower
9. More follicles can be harvested

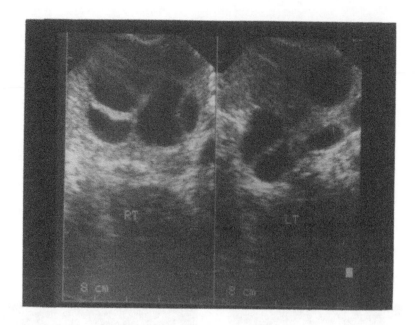

FIGURE 9. The hormonally stimulated right and left ovaries on the day of a planned egg retrieval.

All these factors make TVS the method of choice for follicular maturation studies and egg retrieval.

VII. DIAGNOSIS OF EARLY PREGNANCY

Clearly, the success of an infertility clinic is measured by its pregnancy rate. Therefore, the early diagnosis of a pregnancy is not only a matter of subjective concern for the patient and the entire team providing the care, but it has other important implications that relate to outcome statistics. The rate of spontaneous abortions, ectopic gestations, and multiple pregnancies, which are higher as a result of this treatment, must be carefully tabulated. It is important, therefore, that reliable and earliest possible detection of the pregnancy be made.

TVS makes this possible, since all embryonic structures, including the gestational sac, can be detected at an average of 1 week earlier than by the traditional transabdominal route.[13] By 4 weeks and 2 to 3 d menstrual age (or 16 to 17 d following an embryo transfer), a 6.5-MHz probe can reliably detect a normal intrauterine pregnancy. At this time, the serum levels of β-HCG subunits reach a level of 500 to 600 mIU/ml (first international reference). A 5.0-MHz probe can detect a normal intrauterine pregnancy at a β-HCG level of 800 to 1000 mIU/ml (Figure 11). This is significantly lower than the "discriminatory zone" espoused by Kadar et al.[14] in 1981, or the one advocated by Nyberg et al.[15] in 1985, which are 6500 (first international reference) and 1800 mIU/ml (second international reference), respectively.

Pathological pregnancies such as missed abortions or ectopic gestations (mainly in the tube) can also be diagnosed more successfully and earlier with TVS than with TAS.

VIII. CONCLUSION

TVS is becoming more and more popular in the general field of gynecology, and in infertility in particular. In this paper, the authors attempted to highlight its advantages in the management of the infertile patient. Because the technique confers certain advantages

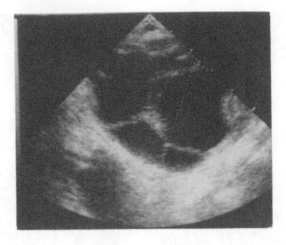

A

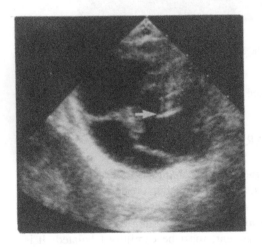

B   C

FIGURE 10.   (A) Four follicles at the time of aspiration, before the needle is inserted. The large follicle aligned with the software-generated "needle path" is the target. (B) The bright echo of the needle tip (arrow) is visible within the follicle. (C) The same follicle is flushed. Note the echogenic (air bubble containing) fluid reexpanding the follicle.

and is relatively simple to master, it seems that it will soon become a major tool for use in institutions and even private offices.

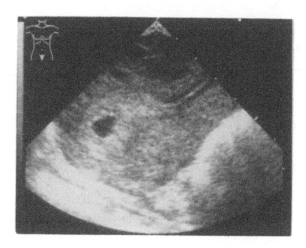

FIGURE 11. A normal intrauterine pregnancy is seen on the longitudinal section of the uterus. Note the gestational sac (8 × 9 mm) within the decidual reaction and the discrete cavity line.

REFERENCES

1. **Lenz, S., Lavritsen, J. G., and Kjellow, M.,** Collection of human oocytes for *in vitro* fertilization by ultrasonically guided follicular puncture, *Lancet,* 1, 1163, 1981.
2. **Hackelöer, B. J., Fleming, R., and Robinson, H. P.,** Correlation of ultrasonic and endocrinologic assessment of human follicular development, *Am. J. Obstet. Gynecol.,* 135, 122, 1979.
3. **Dellenbach, P., Nisand, I., Moreau, L., et al.,** Transvaginal sonographically controlled ovarian follicle puncture for egg retrieval, *Lancet,* 1, 1467, 1986.
4. **Schwimer, S. R., Rothman, C. M., Lebovic, J., et al.,** The effect of ultrasound coupling gels on sperm mortility *in vitro, Fertil. Steril.,* 42(6), 946, 1984.
5. **Timor-Tritsch, I. and Rottem, S., Eds.,** *Transvaginal Sonography,* Elsevier, New York, 1987.
6. **Timor-Tritsch, I. and Rottem, S.,** Transvaginal study of the fallopian tube, *Obstet. Gynecol.,* 70, 426, 1987.
7. **Rottem, S. and Timor-Tritsch, I.,** Think ectopic, in *Transvaginal Sonography,* Timor-Tritsch, I. and Rottem, S., Eds., Elsevier, New York, 1987, 124.
8. **Beck, D., Deutsch, M., and Bronshtein, M.,** The ovary in transvaginal sonography, in *Transvaginal Sonography,* Timor-Tritsch, I. and Rottem, S., Eds., Elsevier, New York, 1987, 58.
9. **Timor-Tritsch, I., Rottem, S., and Thaler, I.,** Review of transvaginal ultrasonography, in *Ultrasound Quarterly,* 6(1), 1, 1988.
10. **Varygas, J. M., Marrs, R. P., Kletzki, D. A., et al.,** Correlation of ovarian follicle size and serum estradiol levels on ovulatory patients following clomiphene citrate for *in vitro* fertilization, *Am. J. Obstet. Gynecol.,* 144, 569, 1982.
11. **Smith, B., Porter, R., Ahuja, K., and Craft, I.,** Ultrasonic assessment of endometrial changes in stimulated cycles in an *in vitro* fertilization and embryo transfer program, *J. In Vitro Fertiliz. Embryo Transf.,* 4, 233, 1984.
12. **Davis, F. A. and Gosink, B. B.,** Fluid in the female pelvis. Cyclic patterns, *J. Ultrasound Med.,* 5, 75, 1986.
13. **Blumenfeld, Z., Rottem, S., Elgali, S., and Timor-Tritsch, I.,** Transvaginal sonographic assessment of early embryonic development, in *Transvaginal Sonography,* Timor-Tritsch, I. and Rottem, S., Eds., Elsevier, New York, 1987, 87.
14. **Kadar, N., DeVore, G., and Romero, R.,** Discriminatory HCG zone. Its use in sonographic evaluation for ectopic pregnancy, *Obstet. Gynecol.,* 58, 156, 1981.
15. **Nyberg, D. A., Filly, R. A., Mahoney, B. S., Monroe, S., Laing, F. C., and Jeffrey, R. B.,** Early gestation-correlation of HCG levels and sonographic identification, *Am. J. Radiol.,* 144, 951, 1985.
16. **Feichtinger, W. and Kemeter, P.,** Ultrasound-guided aspiration of human ovarian follicles for in vitro fertilization, in *Ultrasound Annual 1986,* Founders, R. C. and Hill, M., Eds., Raven Press, New York, 1986, 25.

Chapter 6

IN VITRO FERTILIZATION AND EMBRYO TRANSFER

Asim Kurjak and Marinko Biljan

TABLE OF CONTENTS

I. INTRODUCTION

Since 1977, when Edwards and Steptoe[2] first reported a successful birth following conception outside the human body, a complete new era in the management of human infertility started.

Today, *in vitro* fertilization and embryo transfer (IVF/ET) has become a method of choice in curing infertility in a vast number of couples, where beforehand no suitable way of treatment was available. A rapid development of this method has contributed largely in a more profound understanding of the early stages of human development. This highly sophisticated procedure is a result of the united efforts of biologists, andrologists, embryologists, physiologists, endocrinologists, and a clinical knowledge of all those people dealing with conservative or operative aspects of infertility. Some phases of this procedure are already part of everyday routine, but a recent accumulation of new knowledge has made the procedure even more successful and enabled a widening of its indications.

II. HISTORY OF IVF

Interest in extracorporeal fertilization has a very long and interesting history. After a number of unsuccessful attempts, the first ET in animals was reported in 1890. However, the first scientific results were achieved after the innovation of highly sophisticated laboratory media. In 1959, Chang and co-workers were the first to report fertilization of rabbit ova in artificial conditions. In 1964, Menkin and Rock after long embryological experiments reported successful fertilization of human oocytes in artificial conditions. They proved that *in vitro* fertilization in humans is technically feasible. However, for realization of an *in vitro* fertilization program, a complete team of different specialists was needed. At the beginning of the 1970s, two groups of brilliant scientists started working on the realization of that target. Steptoe and Edwards[2] were the leaders of an Oxford team, while Lopata from Syndey was directing a program in Australia. There were plenty of technical as well as moral and ethical problems to be solved. Lopata was the first to report pregnancy following an *in vitro* program in 1973. Unfortunately, this pregnancy finished with early miscarriage. There was another 5 years and plenty of theoretical and practical work needed before Edwards and Steptoe[2] in 1978 reported the birth of Maria-Luisa, the first baby fertilized outside the human body. They proved that *in vitro* fertilization is feasible in the human and that the result of this process can be a normal and healthy baby.

After them a number of new centers all around the world were opened, and 2 years later, a first Australian "test tube" baby was born; a year later births of artificially conceived babies were delivered in the United States and Western Germany. Up to now, a number of deliveries of artificially conceived babies have been reported from all around the world, and slowly the IVF procedure is becoming a standard routine procedure in advanced gynecological departments.

III. TEAM AND EQUIPMENT FOR THE IVF PROGRAM

Although many simplifications have been introduced recently in the IVF procedure, the process itself is still complicated and therefore is reserved for only highly sophisticated gynecological departments.

The team taking care of the IVF procedure should include several highly motivated specialists and reasonably sophisticated equipment.

A. Laboratory

The most important point of the IVF process is a laboratory equipped to carry complicated tissue cultivations. Conditions in the laboratory should always be under strict control. In the majority of advanced laboratories, the growth of two cellular-stage *in vitro* conceived mice embryos is used for control of the internal environment. In ideal circumstances, embryos develop up to the stage of the blastocyst. The other popular quality of conditions test is a measurement of human spermatozoon survival in the laboratory environment. In acceptable laboratories, spermatozoa manage to survive between 2 and 3 d. As long as the standards cannot be met in the laboratory, IVF procedure should not be put into process.

B. Endocrinologist

The role of the gynecological endocrinologist on the team is essential. He must have advanced knowledge on the stimulation of follicle growth and the oocyte maturation process. He is to decide on the pattern of follicle stimulation suitable for each individual patient. Together with the ultrasonographer he, on the basis of endocrinological parameters, gives an opinion on the best moment for oocyte retrieval. The endocrinologist needs a laboratory equipped to monitor the levels of all relevant hormones in the patient's blood. Especially important is the availability of lutein hormone (LH)-, estrogen-, and progesterone-detecting units. These facilities should be available 24 h/d, 7 d/week.

C. Ultrasonographer

Since Lenz and Lauritsen[26] in 1981 introduced ultrasound-controlled follicle puncture through the full bladder no advanced IVF team could be imagined without the presence of an ultrasonographer trained to follow the growth and maturation of follicles and to collect follicles under ultrasound control. As control of follicular growth is performed every day, (including Saturdays and Sundays) it is advisable to have two ultrasonographers with similar criteria in follicle measurement and endometrium evaluation. A different technique of oocyte retrieval is discussed here. We think that the ultrasonographer should be well trained in all leading techniques. Only those who have a broad knowledge will be able to pick up the most appropriate technique in every situation. For an *in vitro* program, good quality ultrasound equipment is mandatory. It should have at least a reasonable sector and linear high-resolution probe (3.5 Mhz) and puncture imaging facilities. However, the availability of a vaginal probe in many cases makes puncture easier and increases the success rate of the entire process.

D. Embryologist

The embryologist takes care of retrieved cells while they are outside the human body. It is up to him to follow the maturation of retrieved ova and the growth of the early embryo. The embryologist controls and eventually changes the contents of media used in the process.

E. Andrologist

The andrologist prepares the sperm necessary for the fertilization process. He is important in establishing the diagnosis of male infertility and in preparing the sperm concentration most suitable for oocyte fertilization. In large centers, andrologists take care of banks of sperm and together with geneticists decide on the profile of potential sperm donors.

F. Psychologist

The process of *in vitro* fertilization is not only a technically complicated procedure, but also a technique psychologically difficult to handle. Most of the candidates are couples married for a number of years whose long sterility has already changed their psychological stability quite a bit. The procedure itself is quite traumatic. Patients are confronted with plenty of rather unpleasant procedures such as complicated and invasive diagnostic methods and frequent punctures. In addition, the procedure is rather expensive in some countries and patients can afford only a limited number of unsuccessful attempts. Because of all these reasons, we think that the presence of a highly motivated psychologist on the IVF team is advisable. His role should be to calm patients and to enable a healthy approach toward the whole situation.

G. Lawyer

Medical knowledge has been advancing much faster than legal regulations in many countries. A result of this process is that nowadays in many countries there is still no consistent legal or religious policy on IVF procedures. However, in some centers, groups of lawyers interested in the legal aspects of IVF are ready to provide the necessary legal advice to couples involved in IVF procedures. This advice is especially valuable in cases where a third person, such as a surrogate mother or sperm donor, is included in the process of *in vitro* fertilization. In some centers (mostly in those attached to religious institutions), a couple can get a priest's opinion on the intended procedure. In our institution, we formed an ethical committee, a group consisting of an equal number of medical and nonmedical people. Their role is to discuss ethical dilemmas appearing during the IVF procedure.

IV. INDICATIONS

In vitro fertilization is the therapy of choice in cases where no other treatment of infertility can give acceptable results. Therefore, IVF is used to overcome a wide spectrum of infertility-causing factors such as irreparably damaged fallopian tubes (following severe inflammation or ectopic pregnancy), endometriosis, presence of antisperm antibodies registrated in either the circulation or in the genital tract in females and oligospermia, asthenospermia, and presence of antibodies in males.

However, presently IVF is employed most frequently in patients with severely damaged fallopian tubes who have no chance to benefit from the microsurgical treatment.

The male factor is still a rare indication for IVF. Nevertheless, a low fertilization potential resistant to medicamental and surgical therapy could be an indication for the IVF procedure.

The male partner is considered to be infertile in cases where less than 1 ml of sperm, a concentration of less than 20,000,000 spermatozoa per milliliter, motility less than 60%, or morphological abnormality in more than 50% of sperm is recorded. It is an accepted fact that for *in vitro* fertilization no more than a total of 100,000 spermatozoa per oocyte is needed. Furthermore, pregnancy was achieved in cases where ova were subjected to sperm containing less than 30% of motile spermatozoa. These results encourage further employment of that method in the treatment of severe male infertility.

Inasmuch as 10% of infertile couples, complete examination cannot reveal the cause of infertility. Some couples with this uncertain diagnosis could benefit from the IVF fertilization program.

V. SELECTION OF PATIENTS

The selection of patients for the IVF procedure is a rather delicate and complicated task. Therefore, all members of the team should take part in the selection of appropriate candidates.

The following factors should be considered before the patient is included in the IVF program: (1) the patient's age, (2) the quality of ovulation and spermiogenesis, (3) the complete physical and mental health of both partners, and (4) the gynecological status of the female partner.

A. Patient's Age

According to large studies in the literature, it seems that in younger patients the procedure is more successful and safer than in older patients. In patients older than 35 years of age, the possibility of genetic anomalies increases and the rate of successful pregnancies decreases sharply. Moreover, patients of advanced age exhibit a significantly lower response to stimulation of ovulation and an increased rate of early spontaneous abortions. Because of all these factors, women older than 39 years of age should not be included in the IVF procedure. The advanced age of the male partner does not influence the success of the IVF/ET procedure.

B. Quality of Ovulation and Spermiogenesis

In modern regimes, all candidates are stimulated with ovulation-inducing drugs in order to achieve a multiple ovulation, and consecutive higher numbers of transferred embryos. Only 60% of embryos, however, have implantation qualities,[2] and with a larger number of transferred embryos a higher possibility of pregnancy is reached. Recent studies have shown that a pregnancy rate grows proportionally with the number of embryos transferred. However, when the number of transferred embryos exceeds six, no further increase in the pregnancy rate with more transferred embryos can be achieved.[3]

Therefore, the quality of ovarian function and the possibility of induction of multiple ovulation are very important factors influencing the success of the IVF/ET program.

At the beginning of the IVF/ET program, only the couples where the husband had a normal spermiogram were considered for the procedure. Nowadays, with advances in sperm-preparing technology, a successful fertilization with different types of subnormal sperm becomes feasible. The best results are achieved in the cases of oligospermia where the rates of pregnancies do not differ significantly from those in couples with normal spermiograms.[4]

C. Complete Physical and Mental Health of Both Partners

Complete physical and mental health is one of the most important prerogatives for the success of the IVF process. Obesity is a relative contraindication for the procedure. Overweight patients are difficult for ultrasound monitoring and laparoscopic oocyte retrieval. Therefore, obese patients should go on a reductional diet before any other action is considered.

Serious malformations of the uterus as well as abundant intrauterine synechia (Ashermann Syndrome) render the uterus unable to provide a suitable surrounding for the embryo implantation. Therefore, all patients with either malformations or synechias should undergo adequate treatment before the IVF procedure is attempted. Progressive chronic diseases, such as genital tuberculosis and processes involving the liver, lungs, and kidneys, represent a serious contraindication for the procedure. Beginning treatment should be avoided at least 6 months after an onset of serious viral or bacterial diseases in the male partner. In this period, the quality and quantity of sperm are not adequate. Contamination of reproductive organs with *Trichomonas vaginalis* is another factor that sharply decreases the pregnancy rate in the IVF program; therefore, all potential participants in the program should be checked carefully for the presence of this microorganism. Patients undergoing any kind of invasive cytostatic therapy that might interfere with the normal function of the reproductive system are also excluded from the IVF program.

A history of abdominal operations is also a serious contraindication for the IVF procedure. In some cases, laparoscopically guided adhesiolysis can significantly improve the situation. However, in severe cases, especially if the intestina are in adhesions with the genital organs, only ultrasonically guided oocyte retrieval can be performed.

A mental barrier could have an enormous influence on the success of the procedure,[5,6] and the presence of an experienced psychiatrist on the team could be of great benefit.

VI. INITIAL ASSESSMENT OF PARTNERS

Before the patient is considered for the IVF treatment, multiple examinations of the morphology and function of the reproductive tract are performed.

Diagnostic process should start with the standard interview. During conversation, all relevant data in the patient's history should be pointed out. In some centers, the interview is replaced with a rather impersonal but very efficient computerized questionnaire. This type of anamnesis gives more precise results, which are easier to evaluate in any long-term analysis.

After anamnesis, the patient is submitted to a careful gynecological examination. During the examination, all relevant data on the morphology of the reproductive organs and all recognizable pathologies should be notified.

Many important data on the reproductive organs cannot be diagnosed with only a simple palpation. Many more data can be achieved with a precise ultrasound evaluation of the organs of interest. During the ultrasound examination, care is taken with the following data:

1. Size and position of the uterus
2. Size and position of the ovaries
3. Echogenicity of the reproductive organs and surrounding structures in the lower pelvis
4. Detailed description of all ultrasonically observable pathological changes (uterine anomalies, signs of either acute or chronic inflammatory or endometriotic changes, cysts, presence of myomas or other tumors, adhesions, etc.)
5. Evaluation of tubal patency by means of the hydrosonography technique

This basic ultrasound examination is followed by a serial ultrasound examination of the function of the patient's ovaries.[7] The cycle is followed from day 9 of the onset of the menstrual period until ovulation. Every day careful observations on the follicle appearance, size and growth pattern, and comparison with plasma hormone findings are recorded.

After the ultrasonic examination, the postcoital test[8] and spermiogram[9] are evaluated. There is a close correlation between male infertility and sperm concentration less than 20 $\times$ 10^6 spermatozoids per milliliter. However, male infertility is not considered absolute even in cases where a number of spermatozoids do not exceed 5×10^6 spermatozoids per milliliter.[9] Results in treatment of oligospermia are less satisfactory than in cases where impatency of tubes is the causing infertility. However, if a successful embryo transfer with defect sperma is completed, a similar pregnancy rate is expected.[10]

The terminal step in diagnosing infertility is hysterosalpingography and laparoscopy. These are invasive methods reserved for the end of the diagnostic process. Hysterosalpingography could provide valuable information on the uterine cavity, shape, and patency of the fallopian tubes. Laparoscopy, however, enables a close look into the lower pelvis where the extent of extrauterine and extratubal pathology can be observed and some minor adhesiolysis performed. Larger pathological changes will need more extensive operation of adhesiolysis and exposure of patients' ovaries.

If a profound diagnostic process in patients having nonprotected intercourse longer than 3 years fails to spot a definite cause of infertility, a diagnosis of idiopathic infertility is justified. In this small group of patients (according to Zeibekis 11% of all infertility cases[10]), frequently after a long period of infertility an unexpected pregnancy occurs. Considering the fact that advanced age makes pregnancy less possible, if infertility lasts longer than 6 years, a couple qualifies for the IVF program.

Recent advancements in IVF technology have made the treatment of couples with an absolutely sterile partner feasible. There already are a number of reports[11] on fertilization with donor sperm or oocytes, as well as "lending" of the donor uterus, etc. However, all these technically feasible procedures are still the subjects of extensive legal and ethical dilemmas.

VII. PROCEDURE

The IVF procedure consists of several separate, equally important subroutines: (1) stimulation of follicular growth, (2) monitoring of follicular growth, (3) retrieval of oocytes, (4) identification of retrieved ova and evaluation of their maturity, (5) maturation, (6) preparation of sperm form process of fertilization, (7) fertilization, (8) growth and development of fertilized ova, (9) embryo transfer, and (10) posttransferal follow-up.

Only in cases where all these subroutines are correctly performed can the desired result be encountered. Hereunder we will try to describe in short the main point of each of the above-mentioned subroutines. However, the interested reader will find plenty of literature on each subject separately.

A. Stimulation of Follicular Growth

Under normal circumstances, only one oocyte-containing follicle reaches a preovulatory stage. Success of the IVF procedure is in direct correlation with a number of collected oocytes and transferred embryos.[12,13] Substantial effort has been employed to assess a successful induction, which would provide retrieval of the optimal eight to ten oocytes per puncture.

Today, most commonly for induction, a human menopausal gonadotropin (Pergonal, Humergol) and clomiphene citrate in combination with human menopausal gonadotropin (HMG) or in combination with gonadotropin-releasing hormone (Gn-RH) are in use. Pregnancy rates following all types of stimulation are approximately the same, but recent reports show certain advantages of induction with a combination of compounds.[13-15]

1. Clomiphene Chloride + HCG

The mode of action of clomiphene chloride has already been discussed extensively elsewhere in this book. In short, clomiphene most likely reacts with hypothalamic receptors and induces increased production of Gn-RH. From 7 to 10 d after application of clomiphene citrate, ovulation can be expected. Clomiphene is given in standard doses (50 to 100 mg/ d, depending on the body weight) from days 5 to 10 of the cycle. Application of the compound on day 5 enables clomiphene to induce ovaries before selection of the dominant follicle and therefore enables growth of multiple follicles.[16] To overcome frequent atresia of follicles in clomiphene-treated cycles, nowadays in a majority of the centers a dose of 5000 I.U. of human chorionic gonadotropin (HCG) is administrated just before ovulation to provoke ovulation. HCG is administered when follicles reach sizes greater than 19 mm, and when a concentration of estradiol exceeds 300 to 400 pg/ml per follicle.[17]

Even in cycles induced with clomiphene where HCG was administered on time, a significantly lower number of mature follicles, aspirated oocytes, and successful pregnancies than in clomiphene/HMG-[18] or HMG/HCG-stimulated cycles were reported. The reasons for this are, most likely, the inhibition of the hypothalamic function and the local antiestrogenic effect of clomiphene citrate.

2. Clomiphene Citrate + HMG + HCG

This is a very popular scheme that starts with early application of clomide (from day 3 until day 7) and continues with supportive HMG therapy. The dose of HMG is adjusted individually depending on the patient's response to the compound. The indication for HCG adminsitration is follicle size greater than 18 mm with adequate estrogen level.

3. HMG + HCG

Therapy with HMG starts as early as 3 d after the onset of menstruation. Usually a dose of 2 to 3 ampullae are given in a period of 5 d. Further application is adjusted according to ultrasound findings. When a follicle reaches a preovulatory size between 5000 to 10,000 I.U. of HCG is administered. Aspiration of follicles is performed 35 h after application of HCG. A characteristic of this type of stimulation is the always-present numerous follicles, which at the time of aspiration have significantly different sizes. However, in the cycles stimulated according to this protocol in even a smaller number of follicles, mature oocytes are found. A certain improvement in this technique is the introduction of two ampullae of pure follicle-stimulating hormone (FSH) — Fertinum Serano[19] on days 3 and 4 of stimulation. It seems that an increased relation of FSH to LH in these cycles increases the number of aspirated oocytes and the number of clinical pregnancies. In the cycles stimulated with HMH/ FSH/HCG, hyperstimulation with serious consequences is not a rare complication. Therefore, very precise ultrasound monitoring should be performed.

4. Clomiphene Chloride + Gn-RH Intermittent Pulsatile Pump

Recently, a new technique of superovulation in patients undergoing the IVF procedure has been introduced. Initial induction and multiple follicle growth are induced with standard clomiphene citrate and then from day 7 of the cycle an intermittent pulsatile pump that injects 20 μg of Gn-RH is introduced. Preliminary results with this new technique are encouraging, but to evaluate results more data are needed.[20]

B. Monitoring of Follicular Growth

It is a known fact that the best quality oocytes are those retrieved in a narrow period less than 6 h prior to when natural ovulation takes place. Oocytes collected earlier are immature and therefore not suitable for the IVF process. On the other hand, if the retrieval is postponed too long, a natural process of ovulation will expel ova from the ovary to the pouch of Douglas where collection, under normal circumstances, is hardly feasible. Therefore, the prediction of the moment of ovulation is an extremely important detail in the entire IVF procedure. Presently, the growth and maturation of oocytes can be accurately estimated with two methods: ultrasound monitoring and hormonal assay.

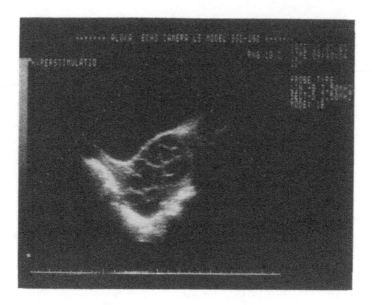

FIGURE 1. Typical ultrasound scan of hyperstimulated ovaries. The ovaries are extremely enlarged and filled with cystic structures.

1. Ultrasound Monitoring of Follicular Growth in the IVF Program

The importance of ultrasound monitoring in the evaluation of normal and pathological cycles has already been described extensively. However, the value of this technique seems to be even much more necessary in the follow-up of superovulatory cycles induced prior to IVF procedures.

In IVF programs in order to achieve an optimal number of mature oocytes, induction of follicles is always massive, beginning early in the cycle. So strong and "unnatural", stimulation always carries a certain risk of hyperstimulation (Figure 1). Unfortunately, unlike in natural cycles, in stimulated ones a good correlation between the size of developing follicles and the plasma concentration of estrogen cannot be established. This is most likely caused by nonsynchronized development of different cohorts of follicles. Also frequently in superovulatory cycles, noncontinuous ("jumping") growth of follicles is observed. This size of preovulatory cycles varies from 19 to 24 mm in clomiphene-stimulated cycles (Figure 2) to 16 to 20 mm in gonadotropin-stimulated cycles (Figure 3).[21,22] The size of the follicle is not in direct correlation with the maturation of the oocyte, and there is no optimum size of the follicle which would guarantee retrieval of the mature oocytes.[23] Some recent investigations, however, show that no pregnancy was achieved with oocytes aspirated from the follicle less than 16 mm in average diameter.[24]

The information mentioned above illustrates that monitoring of the superovulatory cycle is a very complicated job reserved for a very experienced ultrasonographer. Every day during follow-up, the patient should be submitted to ultrasound evaluation of follicular growth, shape, and inside structure as well as measurement of endometrial thickness (Figure 4). These results should be correlated to estrogen and progesterone assays.

We feel that this type of monitoring is the only way to achieve a sophisticated picture of the patient's response to induction and to avoid hypodosage and prevent hyperstimulation.

It is a known fact that both oocyte and spermium are extremely sensitive to any kind of teratogenic agent. Therefore, serious concern for the possible effect of multiple ultrasound examinations on germinative cell maturation and percentage of early pregnancy loss has been expressed many times. However, recent experiments on rats showed that even very prolonged exposition to ultrasound does not affect the number, growth, or fertilization

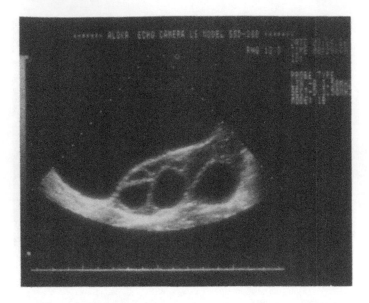

FIGURE 2.   Multiple follicles in the clomiphene-stimulated ovary.

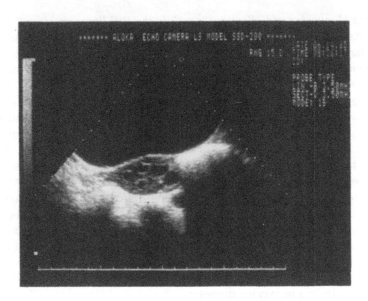

FIGURE 3.   Multiple follicles in the gonadotropin-stimulated ovary.

capability of the rat. The present state-of-the-art is based on experience with hundreds of children born after ultrasound monitoring, and on serious animal experiments; therefore, we can conclude that ultrasound has no visible adverse effect on either subject in reproductive process.

2. Hormonal Signs in Blood and Urine
a. Lutein Hormone

The level of lutein hormone (LH) is the most valuable hormonal parameter in the prediction of ovulation. In the middle of the cycle, only a few hours before ovulation, there is a significant surge of LH concentration in serum. The beginning of the LH surge is the moment

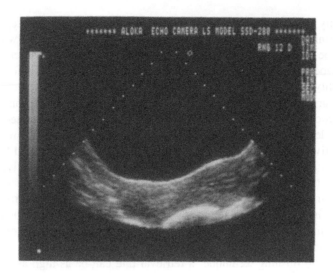

FIGURE 4. Measurement of endometrial thickness. The appearance and structure of the endometrium are reliable signs of the hormonal level in stimulated cycles.

when the concentration of LH exceeds 180% of normal basal values. Ovulation can be expected to take place between 36 and 40 h after the beginning of the LH surge. In order to spot the beginning of the LH surge, its level should be measured every 3 to 6 h.

b. Estradiol

The level of estradiol in serum or total estrogen in urine also can indicate the moment of ovulation. However, the concentration of estrogens is not nearly as precise a sign of ovulation as the level of lutein hormone. Estrogen level is in direct correlation with the size of follicles. At the beginning of the proliferative phase, the level of estrogens is rather low. Rapid increase can be measured 5 to 7 d prior to ovulation. The maximal level is reached before the beginning of the LH surge (approximately 37 h prior to ovulation).

Usually, estrogen is measured regularly a few days prior to the expected ovulation. When the major increase of estrogen concentration is spotted, measurement of the LH should be encountered.

c. Progesterone

Progesterone, a product of luteinized granulosa cells, appears in peripheral circulation only a few hours prior to ovulation. A significant rise in the concentration level can be measured approximately 7 h piror to ovulation. Progesterone is produced inside the follicle and, therefore, can serve as the best indication of follicular and oocytal maturation.

C. Retrieval of Oocytes

1. Ultrasound-Guided Oocyte Retrieval

Ultrasound-guided follicular retrieval was first reported in 1981 by Lenz and Lauritsen.[26] Since then, the technique has been developed tremendously and today, it represents a leading method for oocyte collection in the IVF program.

a. Transvesical Technique

The original approach to the follicles is through the abdominal wall and full urinary bladder. It is basically an outpatient method that requires practically no premedication. However, in some centers to improve the comfort of the patient, 10 mg of Diasepam is administered orally 1 h prior to retrieval.[27] One hour prior to the procedure, the patient is either asked to drink 1 to 1.5 l of water, or the bladder is artificially filled with 200 to 700 ml of normal saline via a Foley catheter until good visualization of the follicles is achieved. Some authors advocate rinsing the bladder with 200 to 300 ml of saline before introduction of the final quantity of saline.[27]

According to our experience, no significant problem with either natural bladder filling or pain during the procedure was experienced.[28,29] Follicles are imaged with a sector transducer wrapped in a sterile bag. To achieve good contact with the patient's skin, repetitive application of disinfective liquid is used. The use of ordinary contact gel should be avoided, as this compound has proved to have an adverse effect on the oocyte.[30] Usually, to collect all oocytes, only one transabdominal puncture is needed. Some authors prior to the puncture apply a local anesthesia with 5 ml of 1% Lidocain.[27] To aspirate oocytes from the follicle, either a simple syringe or disposable mucus aspirator exposed to negative pressure is used. Collected fluid is immediately transferred to the laboratory for the microscopic retrieval of the oocyte. If no oocyte is collected, the follicle is flushed with a medium until the oocyte is retrieved. With the flushing technique, a retrieval rate can be as high as 89 to 91%.

b. Other Techniques

It is sometimes difficult to reach the ovaries or follicles through the bladder. This situation is frequent in cases where the ovaries lie deep in the pouch of Douglas behind the uterus and in obese patients. An additional complication connected with the transabdominal technique is the substantial pain present at each passing through the unanesthetized posterior bladder wall. Furthermore, several authors reported, in spite of premedication, a severe vagal reaction.[31] To avoid this problem, a number of new techniques have been introduced.

c. Perurethral-Transvesical Approach

Campbell and co-workers[32] introduced an interesting modification of the transabdominal-transvesical approach. It is based on their experience that more follicles are aspirated successfully when the angle between the long axis of the ovary and the plane of the needle approximates 90°.

Having a more oblique angle there is a better chance for the needle to miss a follicle as the ovary might rotate and slide away. To overcome this problem, they introduced the perurethral-transvesical approach.

Using this technique, an abdominally positioned nonsterile sector transducer needle embedded in Foley catheter is introduced into a moderately full bladder through the urethra. When in the bladder, the needle is taken out of the catheter and introduced into the follicle through the back wall of the bladder. Campbell and co-workers report a number of advantages of this method over the classic transabdominal approach:

1. According to their experience, the technique is easier to learn.
2. The needle tip is, being almost at right angles to the ultrasound beam, easier to visualize.
3. The transducer does not have to be sterile and a standard contact gel can be used.
4. Conversion to the transvaginal approach is easy.

Of course, use of this technique is not possible in situations where the ovaries are positioned directly behind the uterus, and in rare situations when they are above the fundus of the bladder.

Reported complications are relatively few. In the initial group, neither urinary tract infection nor macrohematuria was observed. An asymptomatic minimal extravasation of urine into the paravesical tissue was observed in only two patients.

d. Transvaginal Approach

Very frequently on the ultrasonograms the ovaries are spotted very low in the pelvis, occupying a position behind the uterus or in a cul-de-sac. Penetration in this location is possible through the posterolateral upper part of the vagina, since according to some new anatomical considerations, the upper part of the vagina in 94% of cases is in direct contact with the pouch of Douglas.[33]

One of the implications of these anatomical data is that the penetration through the posterior vaginal wall will lead safely and directly into the pouch of Douglas without traversing any vital structures. Furthermore, it has been shown that hyperstimulated ovaries in IVF super-ovulatory cycles lie even lower in the pouch of Douglas. Further pressure on the ovaries toward the lower part of the pelvis is employed by the full bladder.

e. Transvaginal Retrieval Monitored with Abdominally Positioned Transducer

All this anatomical and clinical experience led to the development of the idea of follicular retrieval through the upper part of the vagina. Gleicher and co-workers[34] were first to publish on this approach. Soon after the initial report, a number of articles on the technique had been published.

Dellenbach and co-workers[35] developed an interesting modification on the technique. They used a sector scanner positioned on the patient's abdomen to control puncture through the posterior vaginal fornix.[33] To achieve a correct image of the punctured area, an oblique scan through the vagina and ovary was obtained. However, the technique could be used only in patients where the ovaries were not farther than 4 cm away from the posterior vaginal wall. In other cases, Dellenbach proposes a rather peculiar approach through the anterior vaginal wall, and two punctures through the bladder. In this risky method, Dellenbach reports a similar success rate to the one achieved in the ordinary transabdominal approach. In quite a number of procedures, however, inadvertent puncture of the pelvic vein was reported. It seems that a high percentage of serious complications, low retrieval rate, as well as difficulties in obtaining a needle tip during the procedure will prevent wide use of the technique.

f. Follicular Retrieval with Vaginal Probe

In all of the methods mentioned up to now, the technique of full bladder introduced by Donald was employed.[36] Punctures, performed either transabdominally, perurethrally, or transvaginally, were always monitored with the transducer positioned on the abdomen through the full bladder.

An entirely new approach is the introduction of a wide-angled thin vaginal probe, which enables very close contact between the tissues to be punctured and the monitoring system. Such a close relation enables the use of high-frequency, low-penetrating probes (5 and 7.5 MHz), which in turn give fascinating images of the scanning area and precise localization of the needle tip. Because of the elastic character of the vagina, the tip of the probe can be brought close to the ovary by distension of the vaginal fornix. The bowels are clearly visible on the screen and may be removed by rotating and pushing movements of the probe. Using this technique, even ovaries positioned high up in the pelvis can be reached.[36-41] The last but by no means least important advantage of this technique, which contributes to the patient's comfort tremendously, is the fact that the patient does not need a full bladder to have the examination performed.

Considering the possible adverse effects of this technique, one would expect a higher percentage of infection in culture with oocytes obtained transvaginally, and lower pregnancy rate caused by negative effects of Betadine® gel used for disinfection of the vagina. However, so far in the literature, in comparison to other approaches, there is no significant difference in the percentage of infected cultures reported.[36]

In conclusion, it should be said that in the majority of cases, oocyte retrieval for IVF is best accomplished with the aid of a vaginal sector scanner. We believe that this system opens new perspectives for the clinical research approach. In a minor number of cases, where the ovaries are positioned very high in the abdomen, the method of choice still is the classical transabdominal-transvesical approach.

2. Laparoscopy-Guided Oocyte Collection

Laparoscopy is a traditional technique for oocyte retrieval in the IVF process.[1] By means of this technique for oocyte retrieval, successful IVF programs have been established world-wide.

The procedure is performed under total anesthesia. In the operation theater in sterile conditions, through the infraumbilical semilunar incision, Semm's laparoscope is inserted in the abdominal cavity. Before any procedure is started, the abdomen is filled with 2 to 3 l of carbon dioxide. When the sufficient quantity of gas is pumped in, the laparoscope is carefully inserted into the pelvic area. Now under visual control, another suprapubic incision is made and a specially designed trocar is inserted into the abdomen. The role of this instrument is to grab the ovary and enable a precise follicle puncture. Follicular fluid is aspirated with a 25- to 30-cm-long, 1.2- to 1.5-mm-wide aspiration needle. Aspiration is performed under negative pressure ranging between 120 and 140 mmHG. All instruments are kept on the body temperature (37°C). It is wise to aspirate the follicular liquid first from the more mature-looking follicles and only then move to the worse-looking ones. The mature follicle is a blue-pink structure bulging from the ovarian surface. The needle should be inserted through the upper follicular pole into the center of the follicle. Aspiration is discontinued when a complete collapse of the follicle is spotted. The procedure should be performed slowly (at least 30 to 60 s per follicle). Usually larger follicles contain more mature follicles. However, sometimes, even very small follicles can provide excellent oocytes. Therefore, all available follicles should be carefully emptied.

The follicular fluid is examined immediately and if no oocyte is found, the follicle should be flushed and reflushed a few times with suitable medium. Approximately 10% of oocytes are found in flushed material.

In cases where the operation started after ovulation, it is wise to flush the entire pouch of Douglas with 30 to 50 ml of medium. Using this method, it is possible to pick up oocytes from already ruptured follicles. Oocytes collected from the pouch of Douglas can be used in the fertilization process if ovulation was initiated less than 3 hr before retrieval. Laparoscopy enables direct visual control of the aspiration process and therefore more precise manipulation inside the abdomen. Nevertheless, being performed under general anesthesia, laparoscopy carries substantial risks such as cardiac arrhythmias and arrest, bowel lacerations, and severe hemorrhage. Furthermore, during the laparoscopic oocyte collection, the ovarian ligaments and sometimes ovarian tissue are grasped forcefully by the forceps that fix the ovary to enable puncture of the follicles. This in turn can damage the ovarian tissue and its blood supply and adversely affect the luteal progesterone secretion. CO_2 inflation of the abdominal cavity causes a decrease of pH of the follicular fluid[41] and may affect the quality of the oocytes. Transient hyperlactinemia shown during laparoscopy for IVF[42] may interfere with the progesterone level during the luteal phase. The newer methods of retrieval by means of ultrasound have proved to be far less aggressive, require minimal anesthesia, and can be used in practically all patients. In centers where ultrasound retrieval is an established method, no difference in the pregnancy rate between these two methods is visible. In addition, the above-mentioned ultrasound technique can be easily executed as an outpatient, and therefore less expensive, method.

In conclusion, it should be said that since the introduction of ultrasound-guided oocyte recovery, the role of laparoscopy has become of minor importance. With the introduction of the less aggressive, more comfortable technique of transvaginal puncture, it seems that laparoscopy soon will be completely abandoned.

D. Identification of Retrieved Ova and Evaluation of Their Maturity

The fluid collected during follicular puncture is a clear, yellowish liquid with a fairly constant neutral pH ranging between 7.2 and 7.3. The quantity of fluid varies greatly, depending on the size of the punctured follicle.

Immediately upon arrival in the laboratory (a few moments after collection) retrieved fluid is divided into several sterile oval glasses and submitted to careful microscopic examination. The mature complex, consisting of the oocyte and surrounding cumulus oophorus, is quite a large structure floating in the upper layers of the medium, sometimes seen even without the help of a stereoscopic microscope. Naturally, in cases where blood-stained fluid is collected, egg identification, even for a very experienced embryologist, may be a rather difficult and time-consuming task.

The morphology of the cumulus oophorus, corona radiata, and oocyte itself is a fairly good sign of the maturity of collected material.

The mature oocyte is normally found surrounded with transparent cumulus and in highly stretchable intercellular substance. The border of the oocyte, as well as zones pellucida, are clearly distinguishable. Granulosa cells, with characteristic abundant cytoplasm, are found all around the oocyte. Meiotic changes in the mature egg are already completed, and the polar body is expelled out of the cell.

The dysmature cell has no fully formed corona radiata. Granulosa cells are dark and small, forming compact groups around the oocyte.

The third group of cells are athretic cells. These oocytes, due to a number of reasons, ceased their development and have no chance to become fertilized. They are small in size, have a dark cytoplasm, and very rarely have any cells around themselves.

E. Maturation

As soon as the oocyte is spotted in aspirated material, it is transferred to a tube containing 3 ml of media specially prepared for insemination and secured in an incubator.

Preovulatory mature oocytes are kept in an incubator between 3 and 8 h. However, clearly immature ones might need much longer to get into a state acceptable for insemination. Depending on the level of immaturity, these oocytes are kept in an incubator between 24 and 36 h.

When a full morphological maturity is achieved, the oocyte is ready to enter the process of artificial fertilization.

F. Preparation of Sperm for Process of Fertilization

Two hours before insemination, the husband/donor is asked to masturbate into a sterile glass. Immediately upon receipt of the material, the motality and number of spermatozoa are checked. Afterwards, the sperm is washed and centrifuged. Supernatant cellular elements are removed and concentrated sperm is now mixed with medium and submitted for recentrifugation. Supernatant is again taken away and the rest is deposited into an incubator for some 30 to 60 min. Sperm prepared in this way is ready for insemination. Nevertheless, before insemination, rechecking of spermatosoid number and motality is advisable.

G. Fertilization

Between 100,000 and 500,000 motile spermatosoids are added to every mature oocyte. Out of those 500,000 spermatozoa, 500 to 1000 manage to stick to the zone pellucida of the oocyte. Although in natural circumstances such a high number of spermatozoa never get into contact with a single oocyte, up to now statistics show that no significant difference between the number of triploidias resulting from *in vitro* program (4%) and ones spotted in early abortions following natural reproduction could be spotted (8%). To ensure fertilization, the oocyte is kept in insemination medium for not less than 16 to 18 h. Now the microscopic examination in normally fertilized ova should show male and female nuclei and two polar bodies. Sometimes, however, corona radiata cells obstruct a clear view on fertilization and, to get a view of the oocyte, cytoplasm should be removed.

Fertilized ova are now washed and returned in an incubator. The embryos are left to grow until the moment of embryo transfer. Not all of the embryos have the same speed of growth. Between 12 and 28% of fertilized ova do not show any signs of development. The rest of the embryos according to their growth pattern can be divided into two main groups:

1.   Group I. Slow-growing embryos (most frequently originating from immature oocytes) are, 40 to 46 h after insemination, still in the 2- to 3-cells stage. These embryos have a low growing potential, and their rate of implantation is consequently rather low.
2.   Group II. Fast-growing embryos show a dynamic development pattern reaching in 48 h a stadium of 4 to 6 cells. These embryos are much more suitable for embryo transfer, giving high rates of successful pregnancies.

1. Medium for Tissue Cultivation and Embryo Transfer

Several commercially available media are in use with similar success for IVF and growth of the embryo.

Natural conditions in normal fallopian tubes seem to be an ideal medium for fertilized ova, and therefore all artificial media are better or worse copies of the natural liquid in fallopian tubes.

Every week entirely new media should be prepared. Commercially available media are diluted with highly purified water (rate of resistance 10 to 18 M/cm). A precise quantity of calcium lactate, sodium bicarbonate, magnesium sulfate, and penicillium is added. Osmolarity of medium should range between 275 and 280 mOsm/kg with pH between 7.3 and 7.5. Available media contain less potassium and magnesium and more calcium than liquid in the fallopian tubes.

To ameliorate the quality of prepared material, unactivated homologised or fetal serum is added into the medium. For every patient, three different media are to be prepared:

1.   Medium for insemination. Medium is used for oocyte maturation and sperma preparation. It contains between 7.5 and 10% of unactivated serum.
2.   Medium for embryonal growth. It is used for the development and growth of the embryo following insemination. In this medium, between 15 and 20% of serum is added.
3.   Medium for embryo transfer is used mainly for transfer of already developed embryos into the uterus. It contains 75 to 90% of serum.

However, the ideal percentage of sera in media for different purposes is still not generally accepted, and nowadays different laboratories use their own slightly modified "receipts" for media preparations.

The success rate of the entire procedure can be improved if special care is taken of the oocyte extracorporeal surrounding.

For the majority of its life outside the body, the oocyte and early embryo exist in specially prepared incubators. It is more or less generally accepted that the ideal atmosphere inside the incubator should consist of 5% CO_2, 5% O_2, and 90% N_2. The ideal temperature seems to be 37°C. Humidity should be kept between 90 and 95%. All outside procedures should be performed in conditions as near as possible to the ones produced inside the incubator.

There already are available systems that enable water heating of miscroscopes, tubes, tube holders, and other necessary equipment at exactly 37°C.

H. Embryo Transfer

Already grown embryos are picked up from the incubator and transferred back into the natural surrounding of the uterus. This last stage in the IVF procedure is called embryo transfer.

The pregnancy rate resulting from IVF depends on the quality and number of transferred embryos, the acceptability of the uterus to retain embryos and the method of embryo transfer.

It seems that for the success of the entire procedure, most important are normal morphology and reasonably fast growth of the given embryo.

Level of estrogen in peripheral blood could give us quite reliable indices on the readiness of the endometrium to accept the embryo.

There is still plenty of debate on the ideal moment for embryo transfer. In the normal reproductive cycle, the embryo needs approximately 3 d to reach the uterus. In this period, it reaches 12 to 16 cells stadium (morula). Afterwards, it "floats" for another 3 d in the uterine cavity and only then, at the stage of blastula, does it definitely implant into the uterine endometrium. In the IVF process, however, fertilized oocytes are subjected to rather unnatural conditions and therefore behave quite differently than in normal circumstances. Therefore, this means that the natural pattern of implantation should not be copied in IVF programs.

Up to now, plenty of different timing programs for embryo transfer have been reported. Pregnancy was achieved in cases where the oocyte was returned to the uterus immediately after fertilization and in cases where, quite oppositely, embryo transfer took place only a few days after fertilization. However, so far no pregnancy was reported after transfer of fairly advanced embryos (stage of morula or blastula).

According to our experience, it seems that the best embryos for transfer are those at the four- to six-cells stage. Our policy is to transfer all embryos that have a real chance to survive. In some centers, the "surplus" of embryos is frozen and saved for the eventual repeated procedure in one of the next cycles.

Most frequently the embryo transfer technique described by Leeton and co-workers[43] is in use.

Patients are placed in either the dorsal or knee-chest position so that the uterine fundus drops lower than the external cervical os. The tip of the transfer catheter is placed approximately 0.5 to 1 cm from the fundus at the time of the expulsion of embryos. This is determined by either touching the fundus and withdrawing 0.5 to 1 cm, or passing the catheter a distance calculated for the tip to be within 1 cm of the fundus from the previous sounding of the ultrasonic measurement. Embryos are expelled from the catheter in 20 to 40 μl of culture medium. Patients are instructed to remain in the position used for embryo transfer for at least 1 h and to remain in bed for 4 h before leaving the hospital. Even in cases where embryo transfer is performed very carefully, the percentage of its success is still extremely low, making embryo transfer the weakest point in the entire IVF program.

Therefore, a number of new methods have been tried in order to improve the pregnancy rate following embryo transfer. A very interesting idea was introduced by Papp and co-workers.[44] They suggest that an improved pregnancy rate can be achieved if the embryo is tranferred under direct ultrasound control, by means of vaginal probe, directly inside the endometrium.[44] Furthermore, Campbell and co-workers[45] already reported pregnancy following this type of embryo transfer. Additional improvement could be achieved with the injection of embryo embedded in a special kind of soluble sphere. The sphere would protect the embryo for the first several days and enable safe implantation.[45]

Understandably, with higher numbers of transferred embryos, the pregnancy rate increases, Recently, a group[3] from Norfolk proved that in cases where less than six embryos were transferred, a linear correlation between the number of pregnancies achieved and the number of embryos transferred was present. However, transfer of more than six embryos does not significantly influence the pregnancy rate. Naturally, transfer of more than one embryo carries a substantial risk of multiple pregnancy.

I. Posttransferal Follow-Up

A close follow-up of patients after embryo transfer is essential. From 10 to 12 d after embryo transfer, blood samples are obtained. Afterwards, blood samples are collected once a week. Plasma is assayed for progesterone, estradiol, and β-HCG levels by specific radioimmunoassays.[46] Parallel to the hormonal examination, the ultrasonic evaluation of endometrial thickness is estimated. Biochemical pregnancies are diagnosed if an increased β-HCG is found in at least two subsequent blood samples as well as increased thickness of the endometrium, without clinical evidence of pregnancy at the time of ultrasound. If demise is diagnosed after ultrasound detection of heart action, pregnancy is considered to be aborted.

Pregnancies following IVF procedure carry a substantial risk of ectopic implantation. Ironically, the very first pregnancy conceived outside the human body happened to be ectopic.[43] In the literature, the percentage of ectopic pregnancies following IVF procedures varies from 5 to 11%.[48] Since this number is much higher than in the normal population (0.2 to 1.2%), in the IVF program after embryo transfer always when pelvic pain, irregular uterine bleeding, atypical ultrasound examination, and low progesterone and β-HCG are observed, a possible ectopic pregnancy should be considered.

Although there is no evidence that children conceived outside the uterus carry any increased risk of karyotype disorders, in the majority of centers in order to obtain fetal karyotype between 18 and 20 weeks of pregnancy, early amniocentesis is performed. Normal karyotype is the final proof of a successfully completed IVF treatment.

VIII. PRESENT ROLE AND FUTURE OF IVF PROCEDURE

Although the percentage of successful IVF procedures nowadays does not differentiate much from one monitored in natural cycles, there still are plenty of details to be elucidated. However, IVF and embryo transfer presently offer a fair chance for infertile couples to achieve a wanted pregnancy.

It is a known fact that the natural reproductive process in humans has relatively low rates of success. Only 25% of healthy women stay pregnant in the first month of unprotected intercourse, 63% in the first 6 months, and 80% in the first year. Futhermore, another 50% of conceived embryos are aborted before onset of the expected menstrual period. Therefore, out of 100 oocytes, 16 never get fertilized and 15 never manage to implant in the endometrium. Out of 69 implanted embryos, only 39 cases can be expected at term delivery. The reason for such a low pregnancy rate lies, most likely, in the quality of oocytes, spermatozoa, early embryos, and nonadequate receptive endometrium. Some recent studies show that the majority of expulsed embryos have some sort of chromosomal abnormalities. The IVF process unfortunately cannot overcome this natural "inefficiency" of the reproductive process; therefore, a maximal theoretical percentage of successful pregnancies in ideal conditions in cases where only one embryo can be transferred is lower than 10%. Success rates of 25 to 35% can be achieved if more than six embryos are transferred. The cases of multiple pregnancies following IVF have been reported, but they are still very rare. At the present state-of-the-art, 10 to 20% of embryos growing in artificial conditions are fit for implantation. Only 40% of embryos left to develop in artificial conditions manage to reach a stage of blastocyst. Such a low number is most likely the result of the relatively poor quality of media used in the IVF procedure. We can speculate that introduction of new media more similar to the liquid in fallopian tubes will significantly increase the frequency of successful pregnancies and decrease the percentage of spontaneous abortions following artificial fertilization.

The percentage of successful implantations depends largely on the quality and maturity of the retrieved oocytes. Only mature oocytes can grow, fertilize, and implant in the endometrium. Therefore, improvements in the field of stimulation and more precise follicular growth and oocyte maturity monitoring will surely help in increasing successful IVF procedures. It seems that in the very near future, introduction of the intermittent administration of gonadotropin-releasing factors (Gn-RF) as well as induction with combination of a strictly controlled quantity of FSH and LH hormone will give the best results. On the other hand, the vaginal probe will enable the sonographer to receive an almost microscopical view on events inside the ovaries.

The rate of spontaneous abortions following IVF is higher than in normal reproductive cycles. In some of the aborted embryos, chromosomal analysis showed the presence of major chromosomal malformations. However, no significant difference of incidence of chromosomal anomalies could be found between the artificially and "normally" conceived group. Therefore, it seems reasonable to conclude that such a high percentage of spontaneous abortions is the result of the relative "incompetence" of the uterus to accept the inserted embryo. Some authors speculate that the embryo in the early stages of development sends physiological impulses and modifies the quality of receptive mucosa. Of course, in cases of artificial insemination, this inter-reaction cannot be established. Recently, substantial effort has been put into the discovery of the precise mechanism and governing processes in very early pregnancy. These new data might significantly influence the entire procedure.

The introduction of ultrasound opened a new era in the IVF procedure. Quick development in this field enabled scientists to get the real picture on follicle development and to ameliorate diagnosis of approaching ovulation. Moreover, with control of ultrasound, oocyte retrieval becomes an elegant and painless procedure, easy to perform and eventually repeat. Introduction of intracavitary probes (especially the vaginal probe) will in the near future replace all other techniques of oocyte retrieval.[36-41]

Maybe, in the future, more efficient and simpler methods will completely replace the IVF procedure. However, knowledge on the physiology of human reproduction achieved in this field of medicine will remain the milestone of further development.

REFERENCES

1. **Yovich, J. L., Stanger, J. D., Yovich, J. M., and Tuvik, J. M.,** Quality of embryos from in vitro fertilisation, *Lancet,* 2, 457, 1984.
2. **Steptoe, P. C. and Edwards, R. G.,** Birth after the implantation of embryo, *Lancet,* 2, 336, 1978.
3. **Veeck, L.,** Extracorporeal maturation: Norfolk, 1984, *Ann. N.Y. Acad, Sci.,* 442, 357, 1985.
4. **Steptoe, P.,** The selection for in vitro fertilisation and embryo replacement, *Ann. N.Y. Acad. Sci.,* 442, 487, 1985.
5. **Rowland, G. F., Forsey, T., Moss, T. R., Steptoe, P., Hewitt, J., and Darougar, S.,** Failure of in vitro fertilisation and embryo replacement following infection with *Chlomydia trichomonatis, J. In Vitro Fertiliz. Embryo Trans.,* 2, 151, 1985.
6. **Given, J., Jones, G. S., and McMillen, D. L.,** A comparison of personal characteristics between *in vitro* fertilisation patients and other infertile patients, *J. In Vitro Fertiliz. Embryo Transf.,* 2, 49, 1985.
7. **Funduk-Kurjak, B. and Kurjak, A.,** Ultrasound monitoring of follicular maturation and ovulation in normal menstrual cycle and in ovulation induction, *Acta Obstet. Gynecol. Scand.,* 61, 329, 1982.
8. **Naaktgeboren, N., Devroey, P., and Steirteghem, C.,** Successful in vitro fertilisation with sperm cells from men with immune infertility, *Ann. N.Y. Acad. Sci.,* 442, 304, 1985.
9. **Jovich, L., Stanger, J. D., and Yovich, J. M.,** The management of oligospermia infertility by in vitro fertilisation, *Ann. N.Y. Acad. Sci.,* 442, 276, 1985.
10. **Mahadevan, M. M., Leeton, J. F., Trounson, A. O., and Wood, W. C.,** Successful in vitro fertilisation with sperm cells from a man with immune infertility, *Ann. N.Y. Acad. Sci.,* 442, 304, 1985.

11. **Rosenwaks, Z., Lucinda, L., Veek, M. L. T., and Hung-Chiang, L.,** Pregnancy following transfer of in vitro fertilized donated oocytes, *Fertil. Steril.,* 45, 417, 1986.
12. **Kerin, J. F., Warnes, G. M., Quinn, P. J., et al.,** Incidence of multiple pregnancy following human in vitro fertilisation and embryo transfer, *Lancet,* 2, 537, 1986.
13. **Naaktgeboren, N., Devroey, P., Traey, E., Wisanto, A., and Van Steirteghem, A. C.,** Success of in vitro fertilisation and embryo transfer in relation to the causes of infertility, *Acta Eur. Fertil.,* 16, 281, 1985.
14. **Utian, W. H., Goldfard, J. M., and Sheean, L. A.,** Implementation of an in vitro fertilisation programme, *J. In Vitro Fertiliz. Embryo Transf.,* 1, 72, 1984.
15. **Quingley, M. M., Schmidt, C. L., Beauchamp, P. J., Makland, N. F., Berkowitz, A. S., and Wolf, D. P.,** Preliminary experience with combination of clomiphene and variable dosages of menopausal gonadotropins for enhanced follicular recruitment, *J. In Vitro Fertiliz. Embryo Transf.,* 1, 11, 1985.
16. **Marrs, P. R., Vargyas, J. M., Shangold, G. M., and Jee, B.,** The effect of time of initiation of clomiphene citrate on multiple follicle development for human in vitro fertilisation and embryo replacement procedures, *Fertil. Steril.,* 41, 628, 1984.
17. **Trounsen, A. and Conti, A.,** Research in human in vitro fertilisation and embryo transfer, *Br. Med. J.,* 285, 244, 1982.
18. **Quingley, M.,** Selection of agents for luteinized follicular recruitment in an in vitro fertilisation and embryo recruitment program, *Ann. N.Y. Acad. Sci.,* 54, 249, 1985.
19. **Edwards, R. G. and Steptoe, P. C.,** Current status of in vitro fertilisation and implantation of human embryos, *Lancet,* 12, 1265, 1983.
20. **Shaw, R. W., Nduwke, G., Imoedemhe, D., Burford, G., and Chan, R.,** Stimulation of multiple follicular growth for in vitro fertilisation by administration of pulsatile luteinizing hormone-releasing hormone during the mid-follicular phase, *Fertil. Steril.,* 46, 135, 1986.
21. **Smith, D. H., Picker, R. H., Sinosich, M., and Saunders, D. M.,** Assessment of ovulation by ultrasound and estradiol levels during spontaneous and induced cycles, *Fertil. Steril.,* 1980, 333, 1980.
22. **Vargyas, J. M., Marrs, P. R., Kletzky, O. A., and Mishell, D. R.,** Correlation of ultrasound measurement of ovarian follicular size and serum estradiol levels in ovulatory patients following clomiphene citrate for in vitro fertilisation, *Am. J. Obstet. Gynecol.,* 144, 569, 1982.
23. **Buttery, B., Trounson, A., McMaster, R., and Wood, C.,** Evaluation of diagnostic ultrasound as a parameter of follicular development in an in vitro fertilisation program, *Fertil. Steril.,* 39, 458, 1983.
24. **Siebel, M. M., McArdle, C. R., Thompson, I. E, Berger, M. J., and Taymor, M. Z.,** The role of ultrasound in ovulation induction, a critical appraisal, *Fertil. Steril.,* 36, 573, 1981.
25. **Demoulin, A., Bologne, R., Hustin, J., and Lambotte, R.,** Is ultrasound monitoring of follicular growth harmless?, *Ann. N.Y. Acad. Sci.,* 442, 146, 1985.
26. **Lenz, S. and Laurtisen, J. G.,** Ultrasonically guided percutaneous aspiration of human follicles under local anesthesia: a new method of collecting oocytes for in vitro fertilization, *Fertil. Steril.,* 38, 673, 1982.
27. **Lewin, A., Laufer, R., Rabinowitz, E. J., Margalioth, E. J., Bar, I., and Schenker, J. G.,** Ultrasonically guided oocyte collection under local anesthesia: the first choice method for in vitro fertilisation
28. **Kurjak, A., Jurkovic, D., Benic, S., Stilinovic, K., and Funduk, B.,** Interventional ultrasound in gynaecology, in *Recent Advances in Ultrasound Diagnosis,* Vol. 5, Proc. Int. Symp. Recent Adv. Ultrasound Diagnosis, Kurjak, A. and Kosoff, G., Eds., Excerpta Medica, Amsterdam, 1986, 43.
29. **Kurjak, A., Jurkovic, D., Alfirevic, Z., Biljan, M., and Funduk-Kurjak, B.,** Intervencijski ultrazvuk u ginekologiji, in *Intervencijska Radiologija,* Maskovic, J., Boschi, S., and Stanic, I., Eds., Zavod za Radiologiju Opce Bolnice Split, Split, 1986, 153.
30. **Sheean, L. A., Goldfarb, J. J., Kiwi, R., and Utian, W. H.,** Arrest of embryo development by ultrasound coupling gels, *Fertil. Steril.,* 45, 568, 1986.
31. **Dellenbach, P., Nisand, I., Moreau, L., Feger, B., Plumere, C., and Gerlinger, P.,** Transvaginal sonographically controlled follicle puncture for oocyte retrieval, *Fertil. Steril.,* 44, 656, 1985.
32. **Parson, J., Booker, M., Goswamy, R., Akkermans, J., Riddle, Sharma, V., Wilson, L., Whitehead, M., and Campbell, S.,** Oocyte retrieval for in vitro fertilisation by ultrasonically guided needle aspiration via the urethra, *Lancet,* 11, 1985.
33. **Kuhn, R. J. P. and Hollyock, V. E.,** Observations on the anatomy of the rectovaginal pouch and septum, *Obstet. Gynecol.,* 59, 445, 1982.
34. **Gleicher, N., Friberg, J., Fullan, N., Giglia, R. V., Mayden, K., Kesky, T., and Siegel, I.,** Egg retrieval for in vitro fertilisation by sonographically controlled vaginal culdocentesis, *Lancet,* 2, 508, 1983.
35. **Dellenbach, P., Nisand, I., Moreau, L., Feger, B., Plumere, C., Gerlinger, P., Brun, B., and Rumpler, Y.,** Transvaginal sonographically controlled follicle puncture for egg retrieval, *Lancet,* 1, 1467, 1984.
36. **Feichtinger, W. and Kemeter, P.,** Transvaginal sector scan sonography for needle guided transvaginal follicle aspiration and other applications in gynecologic routine and research, *Fertil. Steril.,* 45, 722, 1986.

37. **Kemeter, P. and Feichtinger, W.,** Transvaginal ultrasound guided aspiration of human ovarian follicles for in vitro fertilisation, in *Proceedings of the Sixth Congress of the European Federation of Societies for Ultrasound in Medicine and Biology,* Bondestam, S., Alanen, A., and Jouppila, P., Eds., Finnish Society for Ultrasound in Medicine and Biology, Finland, 1987, 6.

38. **Wikland, M., Andersson, B., Enk, L., and Hammarberg, K.,** Follicle puncture and embryo transfer using vaginal sonography, in *Proceedings of the Sixth Congress of the European Federation of Societies for Ultrasound in Medicine and Biology,* Bondestam, S., Alanen, A., and Jouppila, P., Eds., Finnish Society for Ultrasound in Medicine and Biology, Finland, 1987, 157.

39. **Kurumkaki, H., Koskimies, A. I., and Laatkinainen, T.,** Comparison to three methods of follicle aspiration in IVF programme: transvesical and transvaginal ultrasonographically guided puncture and laparoscopy, in *Proceedings of the Sixth Congress of the European Federation of Societies for Ultrasound in Medicine and Biology,* Bondestam, S., Alanen, A., and Jouppila, P., Eds., Finnish Society for Ultrasound in Medicine and Biology, Finland, 1987, 158.

40. **Sautter, T.,** The ultrasonographically guided oocyte recovery in an IVF and in a gift program, in *Proceedings of the Sixth Congress of the European Federation of Societies for Ultrasound in Medicine and Biology,* Bondestam, S., Alanen, A., and Jouppila, P., Eds., Finnish Society for Ultrasound in Medicine and Biology, Finland, 1987, 159.

41. **Degueldre, M., Puissant, F., Camus, M., Tomberg, A., Phan, T. H., Melot, C., and Leroy, F.,** Effects of carbon dioxide insufflation at laparoscopy of the gas phase in oocyte recovery fluids, Abstr. No. 9 presented at the 3rd World Congr., *In Vitro* Fertilization and Embryo Transfer, Helsinki, Finland.

42. **Soules, M. R., Sutton, G. P., Hammond, C. B., and Haney, A. F.,** Endocrine changes at operation under general anesthesia: reproductive hormone fluctuations in young women, *Fertil. Steril.,* 33, 364, 1980.

43. **Leeton, J., Trounston, A., Jessup, D., and Wood, C.,** The technique for embryo transfer, *Fertil. Steril.,* 38, 156, 1980.

44. **Papp, H.,** unpublished data, 1987.

45. **Campbell, S.,** unpublished data, 1987.

46. **Deutinger, J., Neumark, J., Reinthaller, A., Riss, P., Muller-Tyl, E., Fischl, F., Bieglmayer, C., and Janich, H.,** Pregnancy-specific parameters in early pregnancies after in vitro fertilisation: prediction of the course of pregnancy, *Fertil. Steril.,* 46, 1, 77, 1986.

47. **Steptoe, P. C. and Edwards, R. G.,** Reimplantation of human embryo with subsequent tubal pregnancy, *Lancet,* 1, 88, 1976.

48. **Lopata, A.,** Concepts in human in vitro fertilisation and embryo transfer, *Fertil. Steril.,* 40, 289, 1983.

Chapter 7

INTERVENTIONAL ULTRASOUND IN DIAGNOSIS AND TREATMENT OF FEMALE INFERTILITY

Davor Jurkovic and Asim Kurjak

TABLE OF CONTENTS

I. INTRODUCTION

Ultrasonically guided invasive procedures have been introduced into clinical practice for more than 15 years.[1] In most cases, ultrasound has been used for the guidance of fine needle tissue biopsy of various pathological structures in the abdomen. First attempts have been done with static B-mode scanners, which were sufficient for accurate localization of target tissue, but needle position during the procedure was out of control. The recent introduction of high-resolution real-time equipment overcame this shortcoming and enabled wide expansion of interventional procedures under ultrasound control in numerous fields of clinical medicine.[2-4]

In comparison with other available imaging modalities such as radiography, computed tomography, or nuclear magnetic resonance (NMR), ultrasound has proved to be superior as a puncture guide. Punctures are performed by using small hand-held transducers, and needle point position can be visualized continuously during the procedure. In experienced hands, ultrasonically guided punctures are so safe, accurate, and simple to perform that some authors strongly advocate that an ultrasonically guided biopsy be considered an integral part of the ultrasound examination when additional information about the nature of the tumor is necessary.[5]

Interest for interventional ultrasound in gynecology has increased dramatically after Lenz et al.[6] had described the technique of ultrasonically guided transabdominal aspiration of human oocytes for an *in vitro* fertilization (IVF) program. This technique is now accepted by the majority of authors as an alternative to laparoscopy for collecting oocytes from the ovaries in patients with tubal infertility. Together with the increased diagnostic capabilities of modern ultrasonic equipment, which allows clear visualization of normal and abnormal lesser pelvis anatomy, and the recently developed technique of ultrasound monitoring of follicular growth and ovulation,[7] ultrasonically guided follicular puncture helped to ascertain an important role of diagnostic ultrasound in the diagnosis and management of female infertility. Moreover, it has stimulated development of new interventional techniques under ultrasound control, which are described subsequently as well.

II. COLLECTION OF HUMAN OOCYTES FOR IVF AND EMBRYO TRANSFER (ET) UNDER ULTRASOUND CONTROL

A. Equipment and Staff

Ultrasonically guided follicular punctures should be performed in sterile conditions, but operating room conditions are not required. If a busy IVF program is run, it is advisable to design a special room for oocyte collection which should not be used for other purposes (e.g., routine examinations or monitoring of follicular growth). Laboratory with biologist should be placed next door, because it is of particular importance to provide for easy and continuous communication between the operator and biologist during the puncture. Near-at-hand location of the laboratory helps fast handling of the aspirated oocyte and prevents cooling of aspirated material.

Modern real-time ultrasonic equipment is an absolute prerequisite for successful oocyte collection. Machines should be equipped with either an electronical or preferably a mechanical sector probe. Probe frequency should be 2.5 to 4.0 MHz. Sector probes afford for easy accessibility to the lateral pelvic walls, great maneuverability, and clear visualization of deep-lying structures in the female pelvis. Because of this, sector probes have numerous advantages over large linear array probes, which are not suitable for the successful performance of the procedure. Furthermore, with sector probes it is easier to hit the needle with the incident beam nearer to 90°, when the needle reflects ultrasound better, than if it is hit by the scanner pulses at a grazing angle.

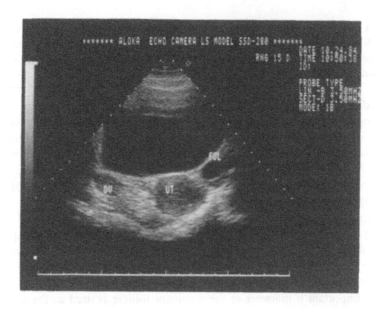

FIGURE 1.   The preovulatory follicle as focused in the marker line on the screen.

The probe should be mounted with a needle-steering device that enables oblique needle steering into the image plane. If a steering device is used, one can predict the needle route upon a marker line on the screen, as the needle is guided via the puncture channel directly into the follicle. This is very convenient when puncture is done by less experienced personnel (Figure 1).

Recently, specially designed high-frequency (5 to 10 MHz) puncture vaginal probes became commercially available (Kretztechnik, Austria; Brüel & Kjaer, Denmark). These sector probes mounted with steering devices are characterized by a large field of view (240 to 270°) and an excellent visualization of pelvic organs.[8] Significant advantages of these probes are shortening of the puncture route and elimination of full bladder technique, which are discussed later on.

From 20- to 25-cm-long stainless-steel needles with stilette should be used. There is no general agreement about the outer diameter of the needle, which enables high recovery rate and minimizes risk of complications. Most groups are using 1.2- to 1.6-mm outer diameter needles with virtually no differences in rate of the successful aspirations and complications. The use of needles with outer diameters of 1.0 mm or less results in decreased oocyte recovery rate and is not justifiable.[9-11]

Aspiration of follicular fluid can be performed either by means of simple plastic syringes with appropriate fitting, or by means of a collection set connection to vacuum aspirator. If plastic syringes are applied, it is important to obtain those that are specially designed for tissue culture. Syringe volume should be at least 10 ml to allow the complete aspiration of the largest follicles. Vacuum aspiration of oocytes does not offer any significant advantage over syringe aspiration, and is relatively more complicated and more expensive. A vacuum aspirator, which builds up and releases the suction pressure immediately, is necessary. The collection set consists of flexible polyethylene connectors that connect the needle and aspirator with a collection tube or flask.

Special attention should be paid to sterilization of the equipment. Gamma rays or dry heat are preferable methods and gas sterilization is not recommended. (For detailed information on handling of the aspirated material, the reader is referred to the comprehensive textbooks that cover this topic.[12,13])

Punctures should be performed by clinicians who possess considerable skill and knowledge of the use of diagnostic ultrasound in gynecology. At least three persons should be trained to perform follicular puncture. Besides an operator, two assistants, preferably nurses, are indispensable for the successful performance of the procedure. The number of trained assistants mostly depends on the organization of the whole IVF program at the department.

B. Preparation of the Patient

In all patients who are scheduled for the IVF program and ultrasonically guided puncture, the presence of active inflammatory disease should be excluded, by the estimation of sedimentation rate, blood cell count, and bacteriological examination of the urine. These examinations should be performed in the pretreatment cycle, and also include analysis of cervical smear and complete semen analysis. Before puncture, the patient should have blood type and coagulation tests checked.

A meticulous ultrasound examination should be made in the beginning of the treatment cycle, before ovarian stimulation therapy is started. This examination is of particular importance to define the ovarian position, to estimate the feasibility of the puncture, and to recognize the eventual presence of intraovarian cysts which can alter patient response to stimulation or later can be misinterpreted for the growing follicles. Detection of intraovarian cysts is very important if diameter of the dominant follicle is used as the basic parameter for HCG application timing. It also helps to avoid puncture of the cysts during follicular puncture. All follicles should be aspirated first to prevent possible contamination of the needle or collecting system with cyst content.

Ultrasound monitoring of follicular growth usually starts on day 9 or 10 of the menstrual cycle and does not depend on the stimulation regimen that is employed. In our own experience, ultrasound monitoring of follicular growth should be performed even in the cases when timing of the puncture is based mostly on hormonal parameter changes. Examinations are performed daily, preferably by the clinician who is supposed to make the puncture in that particular patient. There are two major reasons for such an approach. During several days, the operator becomes familiar with the lesser pelvis anatomy of the patient and is able to acquire a clear three-dimensional impression of the ovarian position and location of each particular follicle within it. He can also accurately define relations between the ovaries and other adjacent pelvic structures like blood vessels, ureters, or fixed bowel loops, which helps in definitive selection of the most appropriate puncture route and avoidance of puncturing any of these structures causing possible complications.

Another benefit is to enable the patient to acquire her own regimen of bladder filling and to get used to the really uncomfortable sense of a full bladder without fear of wretched voiding. Thus, the patients are able to fill the bladder spontaneously before the puncture and it is not necessary to use diuretics or to fill the bladder retrogradely through the urinary catheter. Use of diuretics is not justifiable because of fast bladder filling, which causes bladder overdistension and shortens the time for puncture.

The psychoprophylactic effect of daily examinations should not be neglected. If the operator is willing to explain to the patient the importance of the findings and to illustrate all the details of the procedure, it will help to alleviate the patient's anxiety and improve the patient's cooperation during the puncture in local anesthesia.

C. Ultrasonically Guided Puncture

The patient comes for puncture 30 min before scheduled time and is examined immediately to confirm the presence of the preovulatory follicles. Final preparations for the puncture are then completed. Most patients will tolerate puncture well if only slight sedation and analgesia are applied. Reported premedication is somewhat different between the various centers, but most authors claim that good results can be achieved by intravenous administration of 10 mg of diazepam and 100 mg of pethidin or 30 mg of pentazoizin just before the puncture.

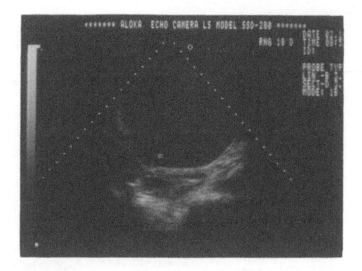

FIGURE 2.   Transverse sonogram illustrating the puncture of the preovulatory follicle under ultrasound control. The needle point is clearly visible within the fluid-filled urinary bladder.

However, these are some patients who may experience intolerable pain during the puncture which can be obviated by doubling the dose. In 3 to 5% of cases, general anesthesia is required.

The sterile gloves have to be rinsed in purified deionized water, and the needle and syringes should be cleaned either by aspiration of culture medium or deionized water.

There are some differences in the final preparation of the patient for the puncture which depend on the selected puncture route and are explained subsequently.

1. Transabdominal-Transvesical Route

This is the first and the most commonly used route for ultrasonically guided oocyte collection. The patient is lying in a supine position and the skin is cleaned with 70% alcohol. Use of various commercially available skin detergents is not recommended. Local anesthetic may be applied to the suprapubic area, but it seems to be of limited value because patients actually do not feel any pain while the needle is progressing through the anterior abdominal wall and bladder. The most painful part of the procedure is penetration into the ovaries, which cannot be eliminated with local anesthesia.

The patient is draped in sterile sheets and the probe is placed in the sterile plastic bag, which makes sterilization of the probe unnecessary. The needle-steering device is then mounted on the probe and appropriate adjustments for fixing and directing the needle should be performed. The first follicle to be punctured is then focused by means of the electronically marked puncture line on the screen. Contact gel is not necessary, but the skin has to be maintained wet with alcohol.

The needle is introduced into the bladder by a short and sharp hand movement. At the same time, the needle point or the whole distal part of the needle is clearly seen on the screen as it follows the guide line. The needle point is then moved slowly to touch the posterior bladder wall and by a short and fast movement pushed into the center of the follicle. The stylet is then withdrawn, and follicular fluid aspirated. If the oocyte has been found in the aspirated fluid, the stylet is put back in place, the needle point withdrawn in the bladder, and the next follicle focused on the screen (Figures 2 to 4A).

Actually, transabdominal ultrasonically guided puncture is a relatively simple procedure and can be performed easily in most cases. In comparison to other ultrasonically guided

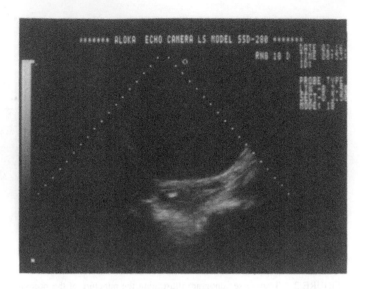

FIGURE 3. Correct placement of the needle point in the center of the follicle.

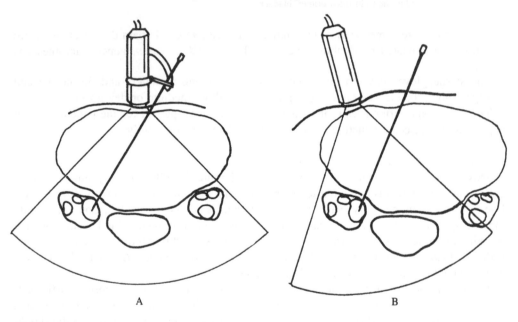

A   B

FIGURE 4. (A) Schematic drawing illustrating the ultrasonically guided follicular puncture. (B) Scheme illustrating the "free hand" follicular puncture. The follicle and needle are visualized simultaneously in the scanning plane. (C) Illustration of the transvaginal follicle puncture. The probe is placed over the lower abdomen of the patient, and the needle and follicle are visualized in one scanning plane. (D) Schematic drawing of the follicle puncture with a transvaginal probe. The probe is mounted with a steering device that facilitates accurate needle guidance. (E) Illustration of the transurethral route for oocyte aspiration. Note that the angle between the needle and the ultrasound beam is almost 90°.

punctures of abdominal structures, the puncture conditions in gynecology are almost ideal. When the needle is placed into the fluid-filled bladder it can be seen exceptionally clearly, which enables easy orientation about its position and direction. Because of this, the transabdominal follicle puncture can be performed in a slightly modified way, i.e., ultrasonically monitored or "free hand" puncture. This technique presumes that the needle-steering device is not used, and the probe and the needle can be moved independently, each held with the other hand (Figure 4B).

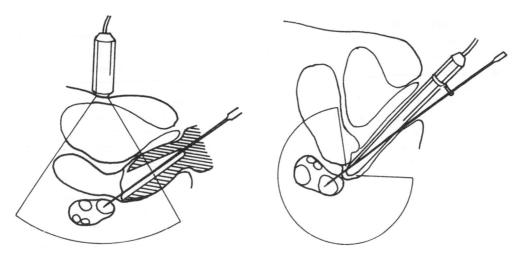

FIGURE 4C.   FIGURE 4D.

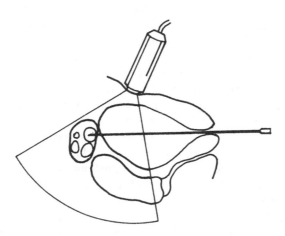

FIGURE 4E.

However, this technique is more difficult to learn, and one should have a clear impression of the scanning plane every moment during the puncture and also be able to move the probe and needle simultaneously, so that the needle never leaves the scanning plane. In comparison to guided puncture, "free hand" puncture offers several important advantages. The operator can move the probe and needle freely and is not limited by the steering device and fixed puncture angle. This provides optimal visualization of any follicle to be punctured and easy avoidance of other structures like thick adhesions or bowel loops. Furthermore, with the "free hand" technique it is possible to puncture follicles in highly positioned ovaries above the top of the bladder, which cannot be reached with the guided technique. The most significant advantage is reduction of the number of abdominal stabs. In guided punctures, because of the needle fixation to the probe, it is necessary to withdraw the needle from the bladder very often to focus the next follicle to be punctured in the guide line. With the "free hand" technique, numerous follicles can be punctured without withdrawal of the needle from the bladder. In most cases, the whole procedure can be completed with only one abdominal stab; rarely are two stabs necessary. This also helps to avoid abdominal scars, which are very often present in IVF patients, or any other unfavorable structures on the patient's skin.

2. Transvaginal Route

The transvaginal route is the second described technique for collecting oocytes for IVF and is used mostly for puncture of the ovaries, which are lying retrouterine, deep in the pouch of Douglas.[14] In this case, it is not possible to reach the ovaries with the transabdominal approach.

Premedication of the patient is the same. Each patient should have a full bladder and is placed in the lithotomy position. There is no need for either abdominal wall or probe sterilization. The vagina is cleaned with an antiseptic solution (Betadine®). The operator holds the probe with one hand and the needle with the other. Local anesthesia of the vaginal wall may be used, but seems not to be necessary. The needle is introduced into the vagina through the speculum. The probe is placed on the lower abdomen and a longitudinal or slightly oblique scan is then employed to visualize the ovary and the needle in the vagina. The lowest-lying follicle should be selected as the initial target. Penetration of the needle through the posterior vaginal fornix into the follicle is continuously monitored. Therefore, transabdominally monitored transvaginal puncture also represents a kind of "free hand" technique, and a steering device is not used (Figure 4C).

The major advantage of this route is easy puncture of low retrouterine-located ovaries, and it is often used combined with the transabdominal-transvesical route. However, as the needle is not passing through the fluid-filled bladder, the visualization of the needle, as well as the estimation of the needle direction, are much more difficult. If the ovaries are placed more than 2 cm from the vaginal fornices, this route should not be employed. In such conditions, the puncture is painful and as the needle is passing through poorly visualized and highly vascularized area, the probability of complications is much higher. Some authors have suggested the use of a transvaginal-transvesical route in such cases. The needle is introduced through the anterior vaginal fornix into the bladder, and then through the posterior bladder wall into the follicle.[15] It is not clear whether such an approach offers any advantage over transabdominal puncture and experience with this technique is very limited.

Recently, introduction of a specially designed vaginal puncture probe opens new possibilities to increase efficiency of ultrasonically guided oocyte collection. The high-frequency sector probe with mounted steering device is introduced into the vagina. Contact with the vaginal wall is provided by an antiseptic gel. Extensible vaginal walls enable placement of the probe close to the ovary and the follicle is focused in the guide line on the screen. This provides for maximal shortening of the puncture route and easy and accurate placement of the needle point into the follicle (Figure 4D).

An important advantage of this technique is elimination of bladder filling and superior visualization of the pelvic anatomy, which also contributes to the accuracy and safety of the puncture. Although the experience with the vaginal probe is still limited,[16] its use is in considerable expansion and probably will be the first method for ultrasonically controlled follicle puncture in the future. Increasing experience will help to elucidate some still controversial points like possibility to puncture extremely high ovaries and incidence of complications.

3. Transurethral Route

The perurethral route for oocyte aspiration has been first described by Parsons et al.[17] in 1985. The patient with a full urinary bladder is also placed in the lithotomy position. The needle is introduced through the urethra into the bladder, and sterilization of the abdominal wall or the probe is unnecessary. There is also no need for local anesthesia. The needle is introduced into the bladder via the urethra by means of a metal introducer with a side longitudinal groove for the needle. After passing the internal orifice of the urethra, the needle is easily separated from the introducer and remains inside the bladder. The introducer is then immediately removed. If the introducer is not available, a self-retaining catheter can serve the purpose of urethral protection during the needle introduction. As in transvaginal puncture, the operator holds the probe with one hand and the needle with the other. By performing a longitudinal scan, the needle is clearly seen inside the fluid-filled bladder. As the angle between the needle and ultrasound beam is almost 90°, this accounts for superior needle visualization and easy orientation about the needle position and direction (Figure 4E).

The transurethral approach is well suited for puncture of relatively high ovaries and is the best method for puncturing the ovaries, which are located above the top of the full bladder. Another advantage is that there are no skin wounds. However, there is always the possibility of urethral injury during the needle introduction.

Moreover, there are no data about whether stretching of the urethra during angulation of the needle towards the lateral pelvic wall can cause long-term consequences on the urethral sphincter competence. Another disadvantage, as indicated in the original report of Parsons et al.,[17] is transient dysuria, which occurs regularly after perurethral puncture.[17]

D. Aspiration of Follicular Fluid

As has been briefly described before, aspiration of follicular fluid is performed by means of plastic syringes or a vacuum aspirator. After the needle point has been placed in the center of the follicle, the stylet is withdrawn, and the needle is connected to the aspirating system. This is an important part of the aspiration procedure, because at this moment follicular fluid can partly escape through the free proximal opening of the needle. The assistant's skill and adequate training are critical at this moment. As aspiration of the follicle starts, its collapse can easily be seen on the screen. Aspiration is completed after complete disappearance of the follicle.

The plastic syringe or culture flask is then immediately sent to the laboratory to check its content for the presence of the oocyte or granulosa cells. The needle is held steadily in the same position within the ovary until, according to the information from the biologist, aspiration of the next follicle or flushing should be attempted. If there is no oocyte in the aspirated fluid, one should attempt flushing of the punctured follicle with heparinized culture medium. The volume of the medium should be equal to the volume of the aspirated follicular fluid. Replacement of the fluid can be seen as the reappearance of the previously disappeared follicle. Heparinized medium is immediately reaspirated. If the oocyte is not found in the first flushing, the procedure can be repeated several times. After successful aspiration of the first follicle, the stylet is put back in place and puncture of the second follicle can start. This technique enables effective prevention of contamination of the needle or collecting system with aspirated urine.

However, a less experienced operator can occasionally find some difficulties in aspiration of the follicle. The most common fault during aspiration is misinterpretation of the reflection of the needle point as its real position. If aspiration is unsuccessful, in spite of apparently clear visualization of the needle point in the center of the follicle, one should try to check the needle poisition by slight tilting of the probe. In most cases, this will result in finding the real needle point position within the wall of the follicle or nearby follicular wall. Misinterpretation of the needle point position is also a major cause of urine aspiration instead of follicular fluid. Unsuccessful aspiration also may occur in a case of proper needle placement into the follicle and usually can be overcome by upside down movement or rotation of the needle.

Needle maneuvering is most important for successful aspiration and an excessive increase of aspirating pressure will not help very much. If a vacuum aspirator is used, the pressure should be sustained at 100 to 120 mm mercury. Increased pressure was also recognized as a cause of oocyte abnormality when it reached 200 mm mercury or more.[18]

As far as aspiration of follicular content is concerned, it should be mentioned that some authors have abandoned follicular flushing by documenting almost the same oocyte recovery rate regardless of flushing.[19] If oocytes have reached full maturity at the time of puncture, they can be found in 92% of cases in the first aspirate.[42] However, there is still the common attitude that flushing is a useful procedure and it is performed regularly by most groups.

E. Management of the Patient after Puncture

After the puncture has been performed through the full urinary bladder, it is important to empty the bladder just after finishing the procedure. Although the patient is able to void spontaneously after the puncture, which has been performed under local anesthesia and sedation, the catheterization of the bladder offers some advantages. It ensures complete emptying of the bladder and easy control of the amount of blood in the urine. Furthermore, complete emptying of the bladder effectively prevents prolonged bleeding, which may occur from the distended bladder wall. If there is significant hematuria, the catheter remains *in situ* and permits continuous control of bleeding.

Prophylactic antibiotic administration, which should be started a day before the puncture, is regularly continued for the next several days.

F. Complications

In approximately 50% of patients after transabdominal-transvesical follicle puncture, small blood clots can be found in the urine after bladder catheterization. This small amount of blood originates usually from the superficial skin vessels. It is found in the urine due to leakage of blood through the needle route, and is more commonly seen in patients who had undergone previous surgery. Blood leakage is seen during the puncture as a stream of echogenic particles which is falling down from the anterior bladder wall. Although it can give the impression of severe bleeding, it is without any significance in most cases. As reported by Lenz,[20] moderate hematuria can be expected in approximately 5% of cases and spontaneously resolves within 24 h.

In a recent report, Feichtinger and Kemeter[8] have analyzed the occurrence of complications after 371 transabdominal-transvesical follicular punctures, and have found 14 patients with moderate hematuria lasting no more than 1 d, which is similar to Lenz's report. Furthermore, they describe seven cases of bowel puncture and two cases of iliac vein puncture which were mistakenly punctured for a follicle but without any complications. In two cases, patients developed cystitis after the puncture, and in three cases, patients complained of severe pain that could not be explained by any pathological finding.

Reported experience with other puncture routes is still too limited to estimate the true risk of complications. However, there is the common impression that, if properly performed, ultrasonically directed follicle puncture can be considered a low-risk procedure, but further comparative trials are required to confirm this.

During the past couple of years, since ultrasonically guided follicular puncture has been introduced into routine clinical practice, there is still the present controversy about the most efficient way of collecting oocytes for IVF. Since the first successful IVF programs were established by using the laparoscopic technique of collecting oocytes, this was adopted by many centers and proven a good and reliable method for the purpose. First reported experience with ultrasonically guided puncture demonstrated less successful results compared to laparoscopy in terms of oocyte recovery rate and number of clinical pregnancies.

However, with increased experience, subsequent reports showed that there is no significant difference in the overall success rate between various centers regardless of the technique of oocyte collection (Table 1). A prospective comparison between laparoscopic and ultrasound group in the same center, as reported by Lewin et al.[24] confirmed these results.

In conclusion, ultrasound has proved to be as effective as laparoscopy for oocyte collection at present, and the oocyte collection technique has no major influence on the final result of

Table 1
OOCYTE RECOVERY RATE PER PUNCTURED FOLLICLE OBTAINED BY LAPAROSCOPY OR ULTRASOUND IN DIFFERENT CENTERS

No. of punctured follicles	Technique	Oocyte recovery (%)	Ref.
1449	Laparoscopy	71	19
806	Laparoscopy	89	21
155	Laparoscopy	59	22
150	Laparoscopy	71	23
29	Laparoscopy	83	24
28	US transvesical	75	24
2086	Laparoscopy	86	25
228	US transvesical	47	25
50	US transvesical	52	9
416	US transvaginal	46	15
	US transvaginal	89	26
150	US perurethral	70	17
623	Laparoscopy	84	8
1568	US transvesical	86	8
323	US vaginal probe	86	8

Note: US, ultrasound.

the procedure, i.e., clinical pregnancy rate. At this point, ultrasonically directed puncture offers some advantages over laparoscopy which are making ultrasound puncture more and more popular.

By performing ultrasonically guided puncture it is possible to organize the IVF program as a complete outpatient procedure. This approach significantly reduces costs and is much more acceptable for the patients. The technique of ultrasonically guided puncture is relatively simple and less invasive compared to laparoscopy. Only slight sedation and analgesia are required, and there rarely is the need for general anesthesia. Besides, it can be easily repeated if successful fertilization does not occur.

III. ULTRASONICALLY GUIDED PUNCTURE OF PELVIC MASSES IN INFERTILE PATIENTS

Although ultrasonically guided transabdominal puncture of various pathological structures in the abdomen for diagnostic and therapeutic purposes is a widely accepted method, there still is controversy regarding ultrasonically guided fine-needle aspiration biopsy of pelvic masses. This method may be particularly helpful in the assessment of patients with discrete ovarian mass which hardly can be classified as being benign or malignant on the basis of ultrasound findings alone[28] Despite reliable experience with aspiration biopsy in other areas of the body, there is widespread scepticism concerning this procedure between gynecologists. The most common arguments against fine-needle biopsy performance in gynecology are fear of the false-negative diagnosis in cases of malignant tumors and possible risk of tumor cell leakage into the peritoneal cavity.[29]

However, present experience does not support these reflections. In a recent report by Smith,[30] results of fine-needle biopsies have been collected from 214 hospitals, mostly from the United States. This includes analysis of over 63,000 punctures. In only 3 cases was needle tract tumor seeding recorded, and in 16 cases infection complicated the procedure. Thus, the approximate occurrence of these complications was 1:21,000 and 1:3333, respectively. It is indicative that only 199 punctures of ovarian tumors were performed among 63,000 punctures and all were made in cases of recurrent malignant disease. There were no reported complications in this group, but it is obviously impossible to speculate about the potential risk of fine-needle biopsy of primary gynecological malignancy on the basis of these data.

Nowadays, ultrasonically guided biopsy of potentially malignant ovarian tumors for diagnostic purposes becomes an important goal and there are several reports that illustrate its usefulness in the preoperative evaluation of gynecological patients. Larsen et al.[31] have reported results of 35 preoperative fine-needle punctures of solid tumors to estimate the reliability of cytological and histological analyses from obtained material. Ultrasonically guided biopsy was performed with a 0.6-mm outer diameter needle for cytology as well as a 0.6-mm Surecut needle for histology. The predictive value of malignant cytology was 88% and histology was 100%. When results of both analyses are added, there are still two cases of false-negative diagnoses in proven ovarian malignancy and two false-positive diagnoses in case of benign conditions. So, there is still place for further refinements of the method, but these results demonstrate significant improvement over previous experience,[32,33] and what is more, ultrasound guidance of the biopsy enables marked reduction of the total number of insufficient punctures.[31]

As far as infertile patients are concerned, fine-needle biopsy of pelvic mass in diagnostic purpose is of less importance. All infertile patients with either clinically or ultrasonically detected pelvic pathology are regularly referred to laparoscopy/laparotomy, which effectively solve diagnostic problems. Besides, these patients, being potentially fertile, are relatively young and are at low risk of malignancy. However, although low, the possibility of malignancy always exists and should not be neglected.

A common problem in infertile patients, particularly those who are to be included in the IVF program, is the presence of usually cystic masses, which originate from either the ovaries or tubes and has been documented previously by laparoscopy or laparotomy. In most cases, these cystic masses represent occluded tubes (hydrosalpinx), large endometriomas, and follicular or theca lutein cysts. There are numerous situations when such structures of known nature are causes of ovarian displacement and may interfere with either successful ovarian stimulation or follicular puncture. In such situations, ultrasonically guided fine-needle puncture of the cyst may be attempted to solve the problem with minimal patient invasion.

There are several reports that evaluate the usefulness of ultrasonically directed puncture of the cystic pelvic mass. DeCrespigny and Robinson,[34] in a series of 30 patients with apparently benign ovarian cysts, have performed successful aspiration of cyst content and have found no malignant cells in the aspirate. They have used the transabdominal-transvesical route with no complications related to the puncture. Of the 17 patients with benign nonendometriotic cysts that were completely aspirated, there was only one recurrent cyst. In the group of seven patients with endometriotic cysts, only one required subsequent surgery.[34] Similar results were also presented by Bovicelli et al.,[35] who used the same technique and found a 29% recurrence rate after simple cyst puncture. Most of the recurrent cysts were endometriotic. There were no observed complications related to the procedure.

In our experience, this procedure has proved to be particularly useful in patients who are scheduled for IVF, and in whom persistent cysts can cause difficulties during the follicular puncture. Ultrasonically guided punctures in these cases are regularly performed during the last week of the cycle preceding the therapeutic cycle. Preparation of the patient is almost the same as for the routine follicular puncture (Table 2).[36] The punctures are performed transvaginally or transabdominally, but if the second route is employed, the puncture technique is slightly modified. To minimize the risk of potential complications, the "double needle" technique is used. The guide needle of 1.2-mm outer diameter is introduced into

Table 2
SELECTION CRITERIA FOR
ULTRASONICALLY GUIDED PUNCTURE OF
CYSTIC PELVIC TUMOR

Ultrasonic criteria	Other criteria
Unilocular cyst	Normal blood cells count
Mean diameter of 4 cm or more	Normal urine
Thin and clear borders	No acute pain present
No internal echoes	No suspected malignancy

the bladder and passed through the posterior bladder wall as close as possible to the wall of the cyst. Then the stylet is removed and a fine biopsy needle with an outer diameter of 0.8 mm is passed through the guide needle into the cyst. The cystic content is then completely aspirated and sent for cytological examination (Figures 5 and 6). We have applied this technique in six patients with laparoscopically proven hydrosalpinx, two patients with large endometriomas in the ovary, and three patients with persistent theca lutein cysts after previous ovarian stimulation without any complication.

In our opinion, the use of the "double needle" technique is particularly beneficial when transvesical puncture of any pelvic pathology is attempted. This approach enables the use of thin biopsy needles (0.9-mm outer diameter or less), which reduce the probability of complications.[30] As the biopsy needle is passing through the guide needle, potential propagation of infection through the needle tract causing urinary infection, or what is much worse, the bladder fistula, is effectively prevented. However, there is always a possibility that one is acutally dealing with malignancy regardless of innocent clinical and ultrasonic signs. Needle tract tumor seeding, although demonstrated in a high percentage of punctures in experimental animals,[37,38] rarely seems to be of clinical importance.[30] By maximal shortening of the biopsy needle route and avoidance of contact between the biopsy needle and urinary bladder, the "double needle" technique is logical for prevention of these complications and their potentially serious clinical consequences.

At present, ultrasonically guided fine-needle puncture of pelvic masses for either diagnostic or therapeutic purposes represents a method that is still under consideration. Further experience is necessary to estimate its real benefits and risks. However, present experience indicates that puncture of benign masses can be safely performed and such a procedure can be easily justified in patients who have undergone numerous diagnostic and therapeutic procedures including laparoscopy/laparatomy.

IV. ULTRASOUND EXAMINATION OF THE UTERUS AND FALLOPIAN TUBES WITH THE HYDROCONTRAST TECHNIQUE

Assessment of uterine morphology and tubal patency is an obligatory step in the evaluation of female infertility. Hysterosalpingography (HSG) is the most commonly used method for this purpose and provides for a clear outline of the inner surface of the uterus and tubal contour. Although HSG is an acceptably accurate method for detection of uterine structural defects and tubal occlusion, it suffers from some important disadvantages, i.e., exposure of patients and staff to ionizing radiation; the use of iodine contrast material, which can cause anaphylactic reaction in an oversensitive patient; and only indirect information about pelvic mass presence can be acquired. Most of these disadvantages are overcome by laparoscopy, which provides for direct visualization of the genital organs, but on the other hand is an invasive procedure and is performed in the operating theater under general anesthesia.

As has been illustrated previously, ultrasound nowadays plays a prominent role in the

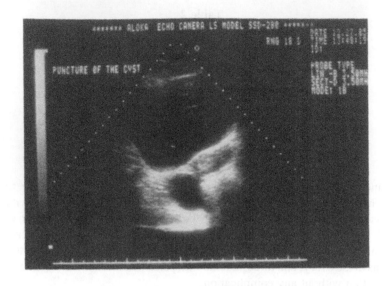

A

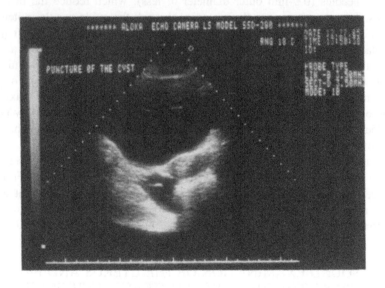

B

FIGURE 5.   Transabdominal-transvesical puncture of a simple ovarian cyst. (A) With the "free hand" technique, the needle point is visualized within the full urinary bladder. (B and C) Position of the needle point is controlled on the screen during aspiration. (D) Complete disappearance of the cyst content after successful aspiration.

assessment of infertile patients. With modern real-time ultrasonic equipment it is possible to visualize numerous anatomical details within the lesser pelvis and to diagnose various pelvic pathology. Being noninvasive and relatively inexpensive, diagnostic ultrasound serves as a logical extension of the clinical examination, and is indicated in the initial evaluation of each gynecological patient.

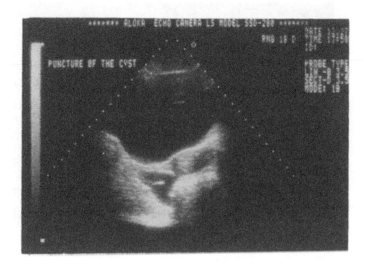

FIGURE 5C.

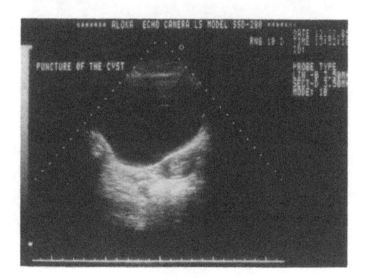

FIGURE 5D.

However, one of the major limitations of ultrasonography in the diagnosis of female infertility is its inability to visualize the fallopian tubes. Although it may be helpful in the diagnosis of gross tubal pathology (tubo-ovarian abscesses or hydrosalpinx), either normal or occluded, but not dilated, tubes cannot be seen.

Recently, experience with the hydocontrast technique has been reported by three groups of authors who unanimously claim its potential value for detection of uterine anomalies and tubal occlusion.[39-41]

The reported technique is more or less the same and includes examination of patients with full urinary bladders with commercially available real-time ultrasonic equipment. After inserting a vaginal speculum, the vagina and cervix are cleaned with antiseptic solution. A suitable cannula is then inserted inside the cervical canal and the speculum is removed. The

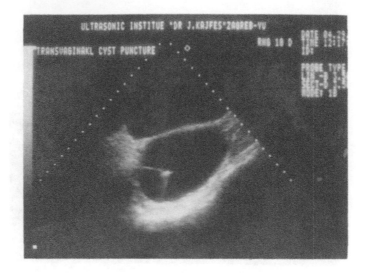

A

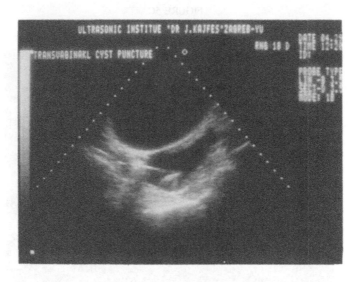

B

FIGURE 6.   Transvaginal puncture of a simple ovarian cyst. (A) The needle
is introduced through the vagina and demonstrated by transabdominal scanning.
(B to D) Aspiration of fluid content results in decreased size of the cyst.

ultrasonic probe is placed over the lower abdomen and a baseline transverse scan at the
level of the middle uterine part is performed. Isotonic sterile saline solution is then injected
into the uterus by means of plastic syringes or pressure pump with pressure not exceeding
80 mm of mercury. It is important to fill the cannula with fluid before instillation to avoid
air bubbles. A diagnostic sign of at least one tube patency is the appearance of free fluid
in the pouch of Douglas.

Richman et al.[39] have found 100% correlation between HSG and the hydrocontrast technique in nine cases of bilateral tubal occlusion. Only in one case, among 25 patients with
at least one patent tube, did ultrasound fail to demonstrate free fluid in the pouch of Douglas,
and an overall accuracy rate of the hydrocontrast technique compared to HSG was 97%.

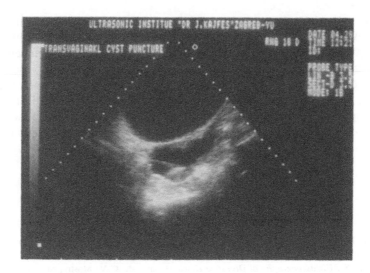

FIGURE 6C.

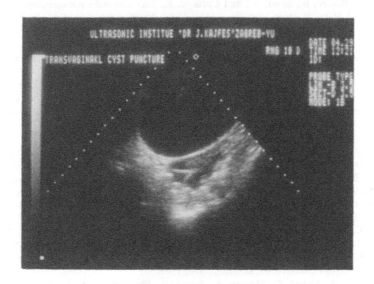

FIGURE 6D.

More detailed study, which included comparison between the hydrocontrast technique, HSG, and laparoscopy, has been reported recently by Randolph et al.[40] In a series of 56 patients with laparoscopically diagnosed bilateral tubal occlusion, there was none with demonstrable fluid in the cul-de-sac. In cases of at least one patent tube, ultrasound failed to diagnose it in five cases. Sensitivity and specificity rates of the ultrasound hydrocontrast technique in establishing the presence of tubal patency were 100 and 91%, respectively. The authors have also tried to identify the side of the patent tube by observation of turbulent fluid flow in the proximal tube or cul-the-sac, but it correlated poorly with laparoscopy. An important observation is that in comparison to laparoscopy, accuracy of HSG in the same group of patients was very similar to the hydrocontrast technique, showing 96% sensitivity and 94% specificity rates.

According to these results, further expansion of the use of diagnostic ultrasound in the diagnosis and management of female infertility can be expected. Such a trend is not surprising, and is the logical consequence of the efforts of clinicians to reduce the use of aggressive invasive methods in the management of patients. This is of particular significance in the management of infertility, because these patients usually undergo numerous diagnostic and therapeutic procedures before final therapeutic success. Although present accuracy of the hydrocontrast technique is lower compared to the other methods for assessment of tubal morphology, it is associated with minimal invasion, preserves the patient from ionizing radiation or operative trauma, and is much safer and less expensive. Further work will define its place among the other ultrasonic methods in the routine investigation of infertility.

REFERENCES

1. **Jensen, F.,** Procedures and principles in ultrasonically guided puncture, in *Interventional Ultrasound,* Holm, H. H. and Kristensen, J. K., Eds., Munksgaard, Copenhagen, 1985, 16.
2. **Weill, F. S.,** *Ultrasonography of Digestive Diseases,* 2nd ed., C.V. Mosby, St. Louis, 1982, 36.
3. **Holm, H. H.,** Interventional ultrasound, in *Recent Advances in Ultrasound Diagnosis,* Vol. 5, Kurjak, A. and Kossoff, G., Eds., Excerpta Medica, Amsterdam, 1986, 1.
4. **Cikes, I., Breyer, B., Ernst, A., and Custovic, F.,** Interventional echocardiography, in *Interventional Ultrasound,* Holm, H. H. and Kristensen, J. K., Eds., Munksgaard, Copenhagen, 1985, 160.
5. **Holm, H. H. and Kristensen, J. K., Eds.,** *Interventional Ultrasound,* Munksgaard, Copenhagen, 1985, 13.
6. **Lenz, S., Lauritsen, J. G., and Kjellow, M.,** Collection of human oocytes for in vitro fertilization by ultrasonically guided follicular puncture, *Lancet,* 1, 1163, 1981.
7. **Hackelöer, B. J., Fleming, R., Robinson, H. P., Adam, A., and Coutts, J.,** Correlation of ultrasonic and endocrine assessment of human follicular development, *Am. J. Obstet. Gynecol.,* 135, 122, 1979.
8. **Feichtinger, W. and Kemeter, P.,** Ultrasound-guided aspiration of human ovarian follicles for in vitro fertilization, in *Ultrasound Annual,* Sanders, R. C. and Hill, M., Eds., Raven Press, New York, 1986, 25.
9. **Lenz, S. and Lauritsen, J. G.,** Ultrasonically guided percutaneous aspiration of human follicles under local anesthesia: a new method of collecting oocytes for in vitro fertilization, *Fertil. Steril.,* 38, 673, 1982.
10. **Renou, P., Trounson, A. O., Wood, C., and Leeton, J. F.,** The collection of human oocytes for in vitro fertilization. I. An instrument for maximizing oocyte recovery rate, *Fertil. Steril.,* 35, 409, 1981.
11. **Lauritsen, J. G., Lindberg, S., and Lenz, S.,** Instruments for human in vitro fertilization and embryo transfer, *Dan. Med. Bull.,* 30, 176, 1983.
12. **Wood, C. and Trounson, A.,** *Clinical In Vitro Fertilization,* Springer-Verlag, Berlin, 1984, 76.
13. **Jones, H. W.,** *In Vitro Fertilization: Norfolk,* Williams & Wilkins, Baltimore, 1986, 1.
14. **Gleicher, N., Friberg, J., and Fullan, N.,** Egg retrieval for in vitro fertilization by sonographically controlled vaginal culdocentesis, *Lancet,* 2, 508, 1983.
15. **Dellenbach, P., Nisand, I., Moreau, L., Feger, B., Plumere, C., and Gerlinger, P.,** Transvaginal sonographically controlled follicle puncture for oocyte retrieval, *Fertil. Steril.,* 44, 656, 1985.
16. **Feichtinger, W. and Kemeter, P.,** Transvaginal sector scan sonography for needle guided transvaginal follicle aspiration and other applications in gynecologic routine and research, *Fertil. Steril.,* 45, 722, 1986.
17. **Parsons, J., Booker, M., Goswamy, R., Akkermans, J., Riddle, A., Sharma, V., Wilson, L., Whitehead, M., and Campbell, S.,** Oocyte retrieval for in vitro fertilization by ultrasonically guided needle aspiration via the urethra, *Lancet,* 1, 1076, 1985.
18. **Lopata, A., Johnaston, I. W. H., Leeton, J. F., Muchnicki, F., Talbot, J. M., and Wood, C.,** Collection of human oocytes at laparoscopy and laparotomy, *Fertil. Steril.,* 25, 1030, 1974.
19. **Rogers, P., Molloy, D., Healy, D., McBain, J., Howlett, D., Bourne, H., Thomas, A., Wood, C., Johnston, I., and Trounson, A.,** Cross-over trial of superovulation protocols from two major in vitro fertilization centers, *Fertil. Steril.,* 46, 424, 1986.
20. **Lenz, S.,** Ultrasonic-guided follicle puncture under local anesthesia, *J. In Vitro Fertiliz. Embryo Transf.* 1, 239, 1984.
21. **Matson, P. L. and Yovich, J. L.,** The treatment of infertility associated with endometriosis by in vitro fertilization, *Fertil. Steril.,* 46, 432, 1986.
22. **Quigley, M. M., Berkowitz, A. S., Gilbert, S. A., and Wolf, D. P.,** Clomiphene citrate in an in vitro fertilization program: hormonal comparisons between 50 and 150 mg daily dosages, *Fertil. Steril.,* 41, 809, 1984.

23. **Lejuene, B., Degueldre, M., Camus, M., Vekemans, M., Opsomer, L., and Leroy, F.,** In vitro fertilization and embryo transfer as related to endogenous luteinizing hormone rise or human chorionic gonadotropin administration, *Fertil. Steril.,* 45, 377, 1986.
24. **Lewin, A., Margalioth, E. J., Rabinovitz, R., and Schenker, J. G.,** Comparative study of ultrasonically guided percutaneous aspiration with local anesthesia and laparoscopic aspiration of follicles in an in vitro fertilization program, *Am. J. Obstet. Gynecol.,* 151, 621, 1985.
25. **Robertson, R. D., Picker, R. H., O'Neill, C., Ferrier, A. J., and Saunders, D. M.,** An experience of laparoscopic and transvesical oocyte retrieval in an in vitro fertilization program, *Fertil. Steril.,* 45, 88, 1986.
26. **Wikland, M. and Hamberger, L.,** Ultrasound in human in vitro fertilization and embryo transfer programme, *J. Fr. Echogr.,* 2, 83, 1984.
27. **Marrs, R. P.,** Does the method of oocyte collection have a major influence on in vitro fertilization?, *Fertil. Steril.,* 46, 193, 1986.
28. **Kurjak, A. and Jurkovic, D.,** The value of ultrasound in the initial assessment of gynecological patients, *Ultrasound Med. Biol.,* 13, 425, 1987.
29. **Jensen, F.,** Puncture of gynecological masses, in *Interventional Ultrasound,* Holm, H. H. and Kristensen, J. K., Eds., Munksgaard, Copenhagen, 1985, 113.
30. **Smith, E. H.,** The hazards of fine-needle aspiration biopsy, *Ultrasound Med. Biol.,* 10, 629, 1984.
31. **Larsen, T., Torp-Pederson, S., Bostofote, E., Sehested, M., and Rank, F.,** Ultrasonically guided fine-needle biopsies for histology and cytology of gynecological tumors, in *Proceedings of the Fourth Meeting of the World Federation for Ultrasound in Medicine and Biology,* Gill, R. W. and Dadd, M. J., Eds., Pergamon Press, Sydney, 1985, 321.
32. **Sevin, B. U., Greening, S. E., Nadji, M., Averette, H. E., and Nordquist, S. R. B.,** Fine-needle aspiration cytology in gynecologic oncology: clinical aspects, *Acta Cytol.,* 23, 277, 1979.
33. **Belinson, J. L., Lynn, J. M., Papillo, J. L., Lee, K., and Korson, R.,** Fine-needle aspiration cytology in the management of gynecologic cancer, *Am. J. Obstet. Gynecol.,* 139, 148, 1981.
34. **DeCrespigny, L. C. and Robinson, H. P.,** Cyst punctures of pelvic lesions, in *Proceedings of the Fourth Meeting of the World Federation for Ultrasound in Medicine and Biology,* Gill, R. W. and Dadd, M. J., Eds., Pergamon Press, Sydney, 1985, 320.
35. **Bovicelli, L., Orsini, L. F., Rizzo, N., Pilu, G., and Gabrielli, S.,** Interventional ultrasound in obstetrics and gynecology, in *Recent Advances in Ultrasound Diagnosis,* Vol. 5, Kurjak, A. and Kossoff, G., Eds., Excerpta Medica, Amsterdam, 1986, 17.
36. **Kurjak, A., Jurkovic, D., Benic, S., Stilinovic, S., and Funduk-Kurjak, B.,** Interventional ultrasound in gynecology, in *Recent Advances in Ultrasound Diagnosis,* Vol. 5, Kurjak, A. and Kossoff, G., Ed., Excerpta Medica, Amsterdam, 1986, 43.
37. **Struve-Christensen, E.,** Iatrogenic dissemination of tumor cells, *Dan. Med. Bull.,* 25, 82, 1978.
38. **Ryd, W., Hagmar, B., and Eriksson, O.,** Local tumor cell seeding by fine-needle aspiration biopsy: a semiquantitative study, *Acta Pathol. Microbiol. Immunol. Scand.,* 91, 17, 1983.
39. **Richman, T. S., Viscomi, G. N., DeCherney, A., Polan, M. L., and Alcebo, L. C.,** Fallopian tube patency assessed by ultrasound following fluid injection, *Radiology,* 152, 507, 1984.
40. **Randolph, J. R., Ying, Y. K., Maier, D. B., Schmidt, C. L., and Riddick, D. H.,** Comparison of real-time ultrasonography, hysterosalpingography and laparoscopy/hysteroscopy in the evaluation of uterine anomalies and tubal patency, *Fertil. Steril.,* 46, 828, 1986.
41. **Mahran, M., Tohamy, S., and Saleh, A.,** Ultrasound examination of the fallopian tubes by the hydro-contrast technique, in *Recent Advances in Ultrasound Diagnosis,* Vol. 4, Kurjak, A. and Kossoff, G., Eds., Excerpta Medica, Amsterdam, 1984, 275.
42. **Kurjak, A.,** unpublished observations.

Chapter 8

ULTRASOUND DOPPLER STUDIES OF BLOOD FLOW IN THE PELVIC VESSELS

Asim Kurjak and Davor Jurkovic

TABLE OF CONTENTS

I. PHYSICAL PRINCIPLES

The measurement of blood flow velocity by ultrasound is based on the Doppler effect, which is named after the Austrian physicist Christian Johann Doppler (1803 to 1853). The Doppler effect implies that the frequency of a sound wave emitted from a stationary source and reflected from a moving interface changes according to the velocity and direction of the moving interface. Movements toward the source will increase the frequency of the reflected waves, and movements away from the source will decrease it. The changes of frequency are directly proportional to the velocity of the moving interface. These changes of frequency are directly proportional to the velocity of the moving interface. This change of frequency is called the Doppler shift, F_D.

If the ultrasound beam is sent towards a blood vessel, the moving erythrocytes will act as reflectors and cause a change of the reflected sound frequency. The Doppler shift is described by the standard equation:

$$F_D = \frac{2F_0 \text{ v } \cos O}{c} \tag{1}$$

where v = velocity of the reflector, F_0 = frequency of the emitted sound, c = velocity of ultrasound in the medium, and O = angle between the insonating sound wave and the direction of the moving reflector.

The Doppler effect can be used to measure mean blood velocity across a vessel area. With two-dimensional ultrasound, all necessary information regarding the angle between vessel direction and insonating sound and the diameter of the vessel can be obtained. Once the standard form of the Doppler equation is used for quantification of blood volume, the total rate of blood flow in the vessel can be calculated easily by multiplying the average velocity by the cross-sectional area of the vessel:

$$Q = \frac{v r^2}{\cos O} \tag{2}$$

where Q = blood flow volume, v = mean blood velocity over the vessel cross-sectional area, r = vessel radius, and O = angle of approach of the Doppler beam to the vessel.

However, quantification of the blood flow can be performed only in the vessels that are demonstrated with ultrasound. The analysis of the blood flow in thin nonvisualized vessels can be based on blood flow velocity waveform analysis. Velocity waveform shows the frequency shift vs. time. It represents maximum Doppler shifts throughout the cardiac cycle, thus reflecting the pulsatile nature of blood flow in arterial vessels. Analysis of flow velocity waveforms is an alternative method of blood flow assessment. The major advantage of this analysis is angle independency and there is no need for simultaneous vessel visualization and diameter measurement.

More than ten indices have been used for velocity waveform analysis. The A/B ratio,[1] resistance index,[2] and pulsatility index[3] are predominately used (Figure 1). According to recently published data,[4] all of those methods provide equally reliable results.

The analysis of the Doppler ultrasound waveform is now widely accepted as a means of studying peripheral arteries.[5] The continuous wave Doppler is commonly used for this purpose. The pulsed wave Doppler, which is depth selective, permits the assessment of deep-lying vessels. Depth selection is achieved by imposing a time delay in the reception of echoes from the transmitted pulse. The position and volume of the sample along the beam axis determine the time delay as well as the length of reception time. The sample position is controlled on a B scan, which can be used alternately with the Doppler system. This

A/B Ratio	Stuart et al. 1980	$\dfrac{A}{B} = \dfrac{\text{peak systole}}{\text{end diastole}}$
Resistance Index	Porcelot 1974	$\dfrac{A - B}{A} = \dfrac{\text{peak systole- end diastole}}{\text{peak systole}}$
Pulsatility Index	Gosling and King 1975	$\dfrac{A - B}{\text{mean}} = \dfrac{\text{peak systole- end diastole}}{\text{mean frequency}}$
Frequency Index Profile	Campbell et al. 1983	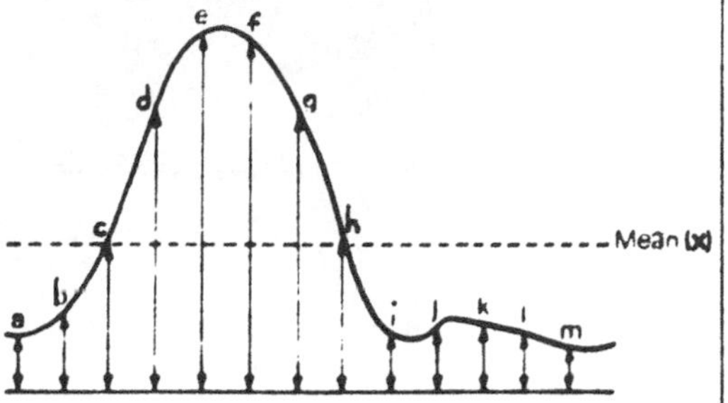 A standard waveform was constructed from the paper strip by measuring the maximum Doppler frequency shift (fd) every 2 mm (0–04s) throughout a cardiac cycle Each value of fd was divided by the mean of all measured frequencies throughout the cardiac cycle and expressed as a percentage of fd (fd/mean fd × 100), called the frequency index profile (FIP), which is, therefore, independent of the angle of insonation and provides a valid basis for comparison between patients

FIGURE 1. Indices used for the examination of the blood flow velocity waveforms.

enables analysis of the signals from any vessel along the beam axis avoiding interactions of signals originating from the other vessels.

II. CHARACTERISTICS OF BLOOD FLOW VELOCITY WAVEFORMS OF THE PELVIC VESSELS

Based on the first ovarian demonstrations of Kratochwil et al.[6] with ultrasound, this method is accepted for visualization of organs and vascular structures in the female pelvis. Thin vessels such as the ovarian artery and vein can be identified as always being close to the ovaries.[7]

By using an ultrasound method combining real-time imaging and pulsed Doppler, it is possible to analyze blood flow in pelvic vessels. The external and internal iliac arteries are easily demonstrated through the full urinary bladder with a B-mode scan. It enables accurate placement of the pulsed Doppler sample over these vessels and records the representative Doppler signal. Flow velocity waveforms of iliac vessels are characterized by high pulsatility, which reflects high flow resistance (Figures 2 and 3). Analysis of Doppler signals enables both quantitative and qualitative analyses of blood flow in iliac arteries. According to Clark,[8] turbulent flow effects that characterize small arterial plaques die out about nine vessel diameters downstream from a stenosis. Because of this, the most important clinical application of blood flow analysis in the iliac arteries is detection of the disease of the aortoiliac segment.

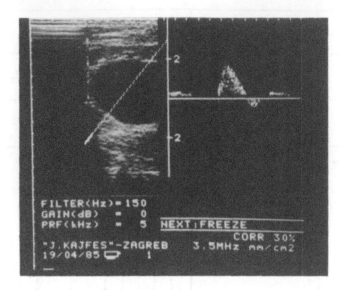

FIGURE 2. B-mode scan through the pelvis with marked sample position (left) and typical external iliac artery velocity waveform demonstrating reverse flow and absent diastolic flow (right).

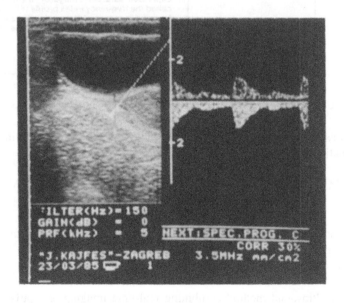

FIGURE 3. Signal from the internal iliac artery (right) showing turbulent flow characteristics and sustained diastolic flow.

Ovarian arteries can be demonstrated with B-scan sonography in 66% of cases. By placing the Doppler sample over the anterior and lateral parts of the ovary, it is possible to obtain signals that represent ovarian blood flow in 55% of nonvisualized ovarian arteries.[9] Flow velocity waveforms from the ovarian arteries have markedly different characteristics compared to those obtained from the iliac arteries (Figures 4 and 5).

The possibility of transabdominal analysis of the ovarian artery velocity waveforms was confirmed by Taylor et al.[10] They have performed invasive studies of pelvic circulation by

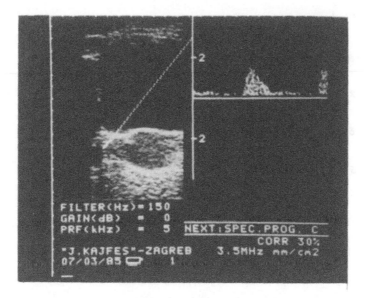

FIGURE 4. Velocity waveform from an active ovary showing sustained diastolic flow (right). Note sample position over the anterior and lateral parts of the ovary (left).

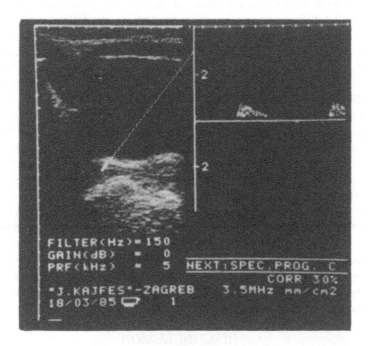

FIGURE 5. Typical low-amplitude signal with absent diastolic flow obtained from the inactive ovary in the menstrual cycle.

applying Doppler transducers directly over the external and internal arteries and ovarian arteries. Characteristics of obtained signals were specific for each vessel under investigation and correlated well with the previous transabdominal studies. An important observation was the significant difference between the signals from two contralateral ovarian arteries, which depended on the side of the developing dominant follicle. Velocity waveforms from the

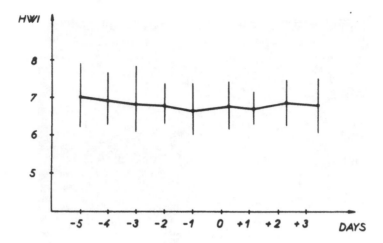

FIGURE 6. Graph illustrating a longitudinal study of ovarian velocity waveforms in 15 normal women with ovulatory cycle. Day 0 represents the day when the dominant follicle disappeared on ultrasound scanning.

artery that supplied the ovary with the dominant follicle revealed sustained diastolic flow and low pulsatility.

Such characteristics of the velocity waveform suggest decreased vascular impedance and increased blood flow. The ovarian artery waveforms obtained from the contralateral side always showed an absence of diastolic flow which implies high vascular impedance in these vessels. Observed differences were present very early in the follicular phase of the cycle when the dominant follicle was not visible on the B-mode scan. This is in agreement with experimental studies, which demonstrated a dense capillary network surrounding the dominant follicle.[11] High vascularization of the dominant follicle is considered to be an important event in the mechanism of follicle selection. This could be an acceptable explanation for significant differences in the ovarian blood supply early in the cycle.

A longitudinal study of ovarian velocity waveforms on the side of the developing follicle was performed recently in our department. Simultaneously with the blood flow study, the monitoring of follicular growth and ovulation was also performed. There were no significant differences in the characteristics of the ovarian blood flow velocity waveforms during the follicular, periovulatory, and early luteal phase of the cycle. Although there were certain indications of marked dilatation of the ovarian artery, caused by midcycle lutein hormone (LH) surge,[12] results of blood flow analysis do not support such statements (Figure 6).

Doppler studies of pelvic circulation also may include assessment of the uterine artery. Signals from the uterine artery at the level of the uterine cervix are almost always recorded and have characteristics similar to the internal iliac artery (Figure 7). Signals from the terminal branches of the uterine artery, which also contribute to the ovarian vascular supply, are inconsistently recorded, and exhibit characteristics similar to ovarian waveforms on the side of the nonfunctioning ovary (Figures 8 and 9).

III. CONCLUSION

The clinical potential of Doppler studies of the pelvic vessels, particularly the ovarian and uterine arteries, remains to be clarified in the future. Doppler studies may provide more sensitive techniques to detect the time when selection of the dominant follicle is completed, to assess the adequacy of follicle development, and to diagnose luteal phase defects.

Unfortunately, at present, it cannot be used for better prediction and more accurate diagnosis of ovulation. Apart from the ovarian physiology assessment, a particularly im-

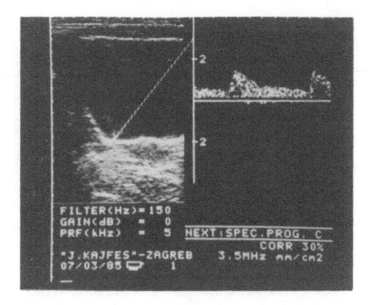

FIGURE 7. Velocity waveform from the uterine artery obtained by placing the Doppler sample close to the uterine cervix.

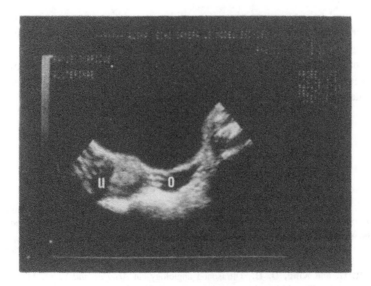

FIGURE 8. Transverse scan showing the terminal branches of the uterine artery reaching the left ovary from its anteromedial aspect (u, uterus; o, ovary).

portant clinical application of blood flow studies might be its use for an early diagnosis of ovarian neoplasms. It can be expected that the presence of very small ovarian tumors might affect the blood flow characteristics in the ovarian artery, but this hypothesis should be confirmed by further extensive research.

Analysis of uterine blood flow has proved to be particularly useful for the detection of various pregnancy complications during the second and third trimesters. Since early changes of blood flow velocity waveforms of uterine arteries were observed in the first trimester of pregnancy,[10] it also may be potentially useful for the detection of an early pregnancy failure.

Recent introduction of a high-frequency transvaginal probe represents an improvement

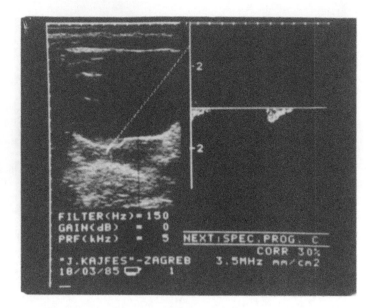

FIGURE 9.   Velocity waveforms obtained from the previously visualized terminal branches of the uterine artery.

over transabdominal pelvic sonography. It provides a superior visualization of anatomical details and more accurate detection of pelvic pathology.[13] Initial experience of Doppler studies with vaginal probes suggests that improvements also may be expected in this field.[14] Close placement of the probe to the vessel under investigation overcomes some physical limitations posed by the large distance between the probe and the vessel. Further work will show to what degree the predictions are truthful and valuable.

REFERENCES

1. **Gosling, R. G.,** Extraction of physiological information from spectrum analysed Doppler-shifted continuous wave ultrasound signal obtained non-invasively from the arterial tree, in *IEE Medical Monographics,* Hill, D. M. and Watson, B. W., Eds., Peter Peregrinus, London, 1976, 73.
2. **Pourcelot, L.,** Application cliniques de l'examen Doppler transcutane, in *Velocimetric Ultrasoner Doppler,* Peronnean, P., Ed., Inserm, Paris, 1974, 625.
3. **Gosling, R. G. and King, D. H.,** Ultrasound angiology, in *Arteries and Veins,* Marcus, A. W. and Adamson, L., Eds., Churchill Livingstone, Edinburgh, 1975, 61.
4. **Mulders, L. G. M., Wijn, P. F. F., Jonsma, H. W., and Heni, R. R.,** A comparative study of three indices of umbilical blood flow in relation to the prediction of growth retardation, *J. Perinat. Med.,* 15, 3, 1987.
5. **Johnston, K. W. and Taraschuk, I.,** Validation of the role of pulsatility index in quantitation of the severity of peripheral arterial occlusive disease, *Am. J. Surg.,* 131, 295, 1976.
6. **Kratochwil, A., Urban, G., and Freidreich, F.,** Ultrasonic tomography of the ovaries, *Ann. Chir. Gynecol. Fenn.,* 6, 211, 1972.
7. **Hackelöer, B. J. and Nitschke-Dabelstein, S.,** Ovarian imaging by ultrasound: an attempt to define a reference plane, *J. Clin. Ultrasound,* 9, 275, 1980.
8. **Clark, C.,** The propagation of turbulence produced by a stenosis, *J. Biomech.,* 13, 591, 1980.
9. **Kurjak, A. and Jurkovic, D.,** New ultrasonic technique for assessing circulation in the female pelvis, in *Recent Advances in Ultrasound Diagnosis,* Vol. 5, Kurjak, A. and Kossoff, G., Eds., Excerpta Medica, Amsterdam, 1986, 198.

10. **Taylor, K. J. W., Burns, P. N., Wells, P. N. T., Conway, D. I., and Hull, M. G. R.,** Ultrasound Doppler flow studies of the ovarian and uterine arteries, *Br. J. Obstet. Gynaecol.,* 92, 240, 1985.
11. **Zeleznik, A. J.,** Factors governing the selection of the preovulatory follicle in the rhesus monkey, in *Follicular Maturation and Ovulation,* Rolland, R., van Hall, E. V., Hillier, S. G., McNatty, K. P., and Schoemaker, J., Eds., Excerpta Medica, Amsterdam, 1982, 37.
12. **Trimor-Tritsch, I. E. and Rottem, S.,** The appearance of the early abnormal pregnancy by a 6.5 MHz transvaginal probe, in *Proceedings of the Sixth Congress of the Europian Federation of Societies of Ultrasound in Medicine and Biology,* Bondestam, S., Alanen, A., and Jouppila, P., Eds., Euroson, Helsinki, 1987, 208.

Chapter 9

SONOGRAPHY IN MALE INFERTILITY

Zeljko Fuchkar

TABLE OF CONTENTS

I. INTRODUCTION

The adequate clinical management of infertility includes the male partner examination. The male partner is responsible for infertility in up to 50% of cases. Most often, male infertility is due to obstructive and/or inflammatory processes affecting any part of the urogenital tract and hormonal state depletion. These abnormalities result in a spermatogenic defect (95%) and most of these patients produce sperm in some quantity accompanied by defects in the spermatozoid feature, motility, and number.

Oligospermia, which is defined as the reduced number of sperm cells, less than 20,000,000 spermatozoids per milliliter, is the most common finding. The etiology of oligospermia could be

1. Congenital (Klinefelter's syndrome, defects of seminiferous tubules, kryptorchism)
2. Hormonal (hypopituitarism)
3. Infectious (mumps orchitis, various bacterial infections of the testis, epididymis, prostate, and seminal vesicles)
4. Traumatic

By means of urological diagnostic methods, as well as evaluation, cystourethroscopy, deferentovasography, and testicular biopsy, it is possible to differentiate between hormonal/congenital oligospermia.

Azoospermia, i.e., the absence of sperm cells in ejaculate, often results from occlusion of the sperm transport mechanism, and is caused by various bacterial infections, traumatic injuries, or congenital anomalies (absence of vasa and/or seminal vesicles). In some instances, infertility may be generated by mechanical factors in the presence of normal spermatogenesis:

1. After surgical procedures (vasal trauma during herniorrhaphy or orchidopexy, bilateral vasectomy for medical purposes or elective sterilization, some pelvic operations) where the transport system is directly damaged
2. After surgery of the prostatic urethra and vesical neck where retrograde intravesical ejaculation is often present, and caused by inability of vesical neck closure

Invasive methods for the diagnosis of male infertility (endoscopy, puncture) may be associated with significant complications, as are infections, bleeding, and postoperative strictures. This fact offers a direction for the use of noninvasive methods in the management of these patients. Ultrasound, being an entirely noninvasive and safe method has been used widely in clinical practice during the past years.

Diagnostic accuracy of ultrasound in the field of male infertility has been reported extensively.

II. PROSTATE

Acute and, particularly, chronic prostatitis may induce fibrosis and stricture of one or both vasa. The capsule and prostatic parenchyma of normal prostate are easily demonstrated by suprapubic and transrectal sonography. Prostatic volumetry by means of ultrasound[5] is helpful in the follow-up of conservative treatment of prostatic inflammatory diseases. The normal prostatic capsule is visible as a continuous, symmetrical outline of variable shape. Internal echoes are homogeneous in distribution, but very often small areas of varying intensity with low gain setting can be noticed. Urethra and periurethral structures can be seen as small hyperechogenic areas within the prostatic parenchyma (Figure 1).

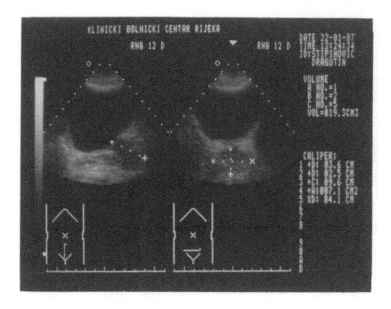

FIGURE 1. Suprapubic longitudinal and transversal sector scans of the normal prostate with calculation of the prostatic volume.

A. Acute Prostatitis

Typical ultrasonic characteristics are easily demonstrated by the performing scan. The prostate is enlarged, swollen, and hypoechogenic. Successful conservative treatment results in the sonographic finding of normal gland size. The presence of postinflammatory fibrotic tissue is occasionally seen as increased focal echogenicity.

B. Chronic Prostatitis

Chronic prostatitis is marked by unusual sonographic findings. The prostate is filled with the hyperechoic areas, and exacerbation of inflammation is seen as the reappearance of small hypoechogenic areas. Such a sonographic picture denotes chronic suppurative prostatitis, and if it is caused by coliform bacteria, then it may result in decreased sperm motility. Chronic prostatitis and prostatic cancer are often indistinguishable on the basis of sonographic examination alone.[2,6]

Capsular irregularity or partial prostatic enlargement should arouse suspicion of the presence of malignancy. Progression of focal lesions is an indication of sonographically guided prostatic biopsy (Figures 2 and 3).[7]

Spreading of the prostatic infection into the vasa deferentia may induce fibrosis, stricture, or total occlusion of one or both vasoprostatic connections.

C. Prostatic Abscess

Prostatic abscess is the final stage of the focal infection. Posteriorly placed abscesses, with huge fibrotic capsula, can occlude the vasa deferentia, or spread infection and secondary strictures.

Operative treatment (transurethral or transrectal) of prostatic abscess could have some sequelae (stricture or occlusion of the vasa deferentia, propagation of bacterial infection with deferentitis, and/ or orchiepididymitis) with final azoo- or oligospermia (Figures 4 and 5).

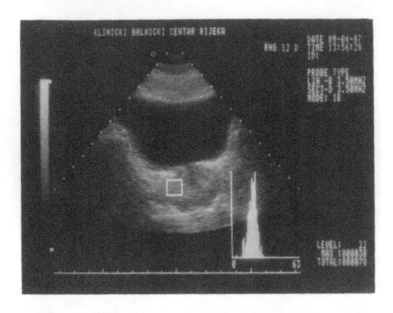

FIGURE 2. Suprapubic transversal sector scan of chronic prostatitis with histogram presentation.

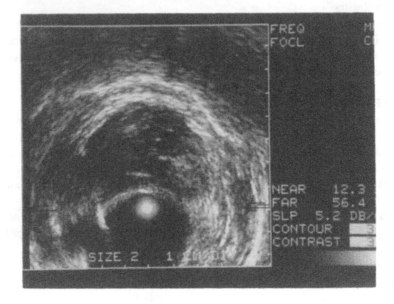

FIGURE 3. Transrectal transverse scan of chronic prostatitis.

III. SEMINAL VESICLES

The seminal vesicles are important in the elaboration of the seminal plasma, and their secretions form up to 80% of the total ejaculate. Abnormal fructose metabolism in the seminal vesicle may contribute to the inadequate storage capacity and diminished number of spermatozoa available for fertilization. Decreased volume capacity of seminal vesicles in chronic inflammation can lead to relative infertility with normal spermiogenesis. Residual fibrotic tissue, after acute vesiculitis, can result in stenosis or stricture of the vesiculoprostatic segment. On the longitudinal suprapubic scan (Figure 4), the seminal vesicles appear as

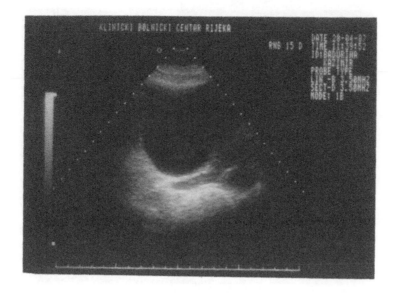

FIGURE 4. Suprapubic longitudinal sector scan of a prostate with a posteriorly placed abscess and seminal vesicle.

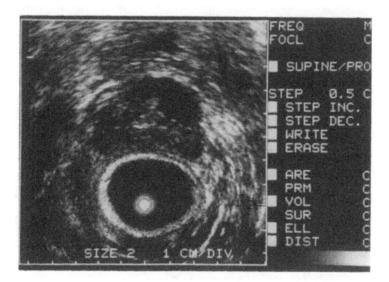

FIGURE 5. Transrectal transverse scan of the medial portion of the normal prostatic tissue with abscess formation of the left prostatic lobe.

small ovoid hypoechoic formations, placed cranially to the prostate. Transversal scans show two small ovoid hypoechogenic areas near the posterior detrusor wall. Sometimes they have asymmetric features, but echogenicity must be equal. The presence of internal echoes and hyper- or hypoechogenicity of the capsule are the pathological findings. Correct sonographic diagnosis of seminal vesicle diseases can be established in 92% of patients with the transrectal approach, while suprapubic sonography enables diagnosis[8] in 68% patients. The technique of sonographic exploration and volumetry also has been described.[1,8,9] Congenital absence of the vas and seminal vesicles may occur as an isolated anatomical defect (Figures 6 to 8).

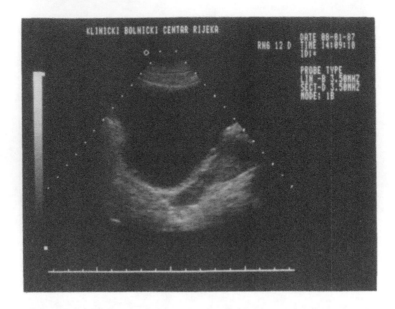

FIGURE 6.   Suprapubic longitudinal sector scan of a normal prostate and seminal vesicle.

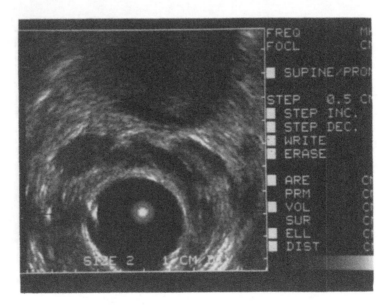

FIGURE 7.   Transrectal transverse scan of both seminal vesicles (normal sonographic feature).

A. Acute Vesiculitis

During the routine urological examination, acute vesiculitis cannot be detected easily, and invasive radiographic technique or cystoscopy has to be employed. In most cases, acute vesiculitis is accompanied by acute prostatitis (Figure 9). The affected seminal vesicle is enlarged, swollen, and hypoechogenic compared to the contralateral one. The boundaries are not clearly defined because of the periseminal edema. The effects of therapy could be followed by repeated sonographic examinations (Figures 10 and 11).

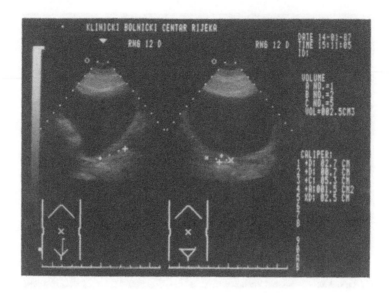

FIGURE 8. Longitudinal sector scan of normal seminal vesicles with volume calculation.

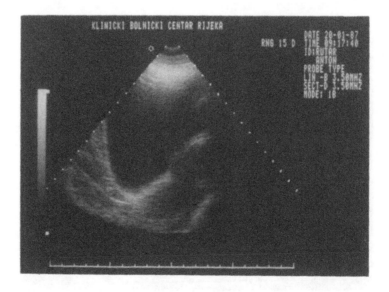

FIGURE 9. Suprapubic longitudinal sector scan of acute prostatitis and acute vesiculitis.

B. Chronic Vesiculitis

Ultrasound diagnosis of chronic vesiculitis suffers from significant limitations, because of similarity to malignant disease appearance. Variability of sonographic finding depends on heterogenicity of pathomorphological changes in chronic inflammatory processes, i.e., fibrosis, areas of recurrent active infection, scars, and changes in vascularization. Antibiotic therapy, based on antibiogram, is sometimes effective therapy for chronic infection and could result in complete recovery. Drug injection into the seminal vesicles, under sonographic guidance (antibiotics, corticosteroids), is an effective treatment of the disease in approximately 2/3 of cases. The seminal vesicles were larger in patients with a previous diagnosis

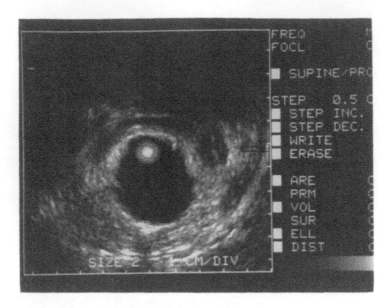

FIGURE 10.   Transrectal transverse scan of right acute vesiculitis (note the asymmetry of the seminal vesicles).

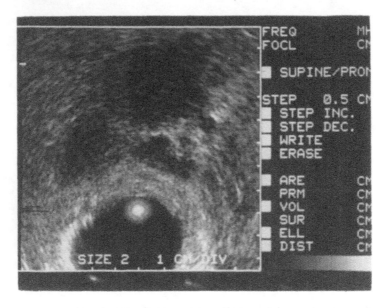

FIGURE 11.   Transrectal transversal scan of the same patient as in Figure 10 after conservative treatment of acute prostatitis.

of prostatitis. Infrequently, the seminal vesicles are the site of cysts,[10] tumors, or congenital malformations.[11] Stone formations within the seminal vesicles are rare (Figures 12 and 13).

IV. SPERMATIC CORD (VASA DEFERENTIA)

Acute epididymitis is a frequent urological diagnosis. Spreading of infection into the spermatic cord and perideferential tissue may result in fibrosis and stricture or total occlusion of one or both vasa. This is particularly common in tuberculous and gonococcal infections.

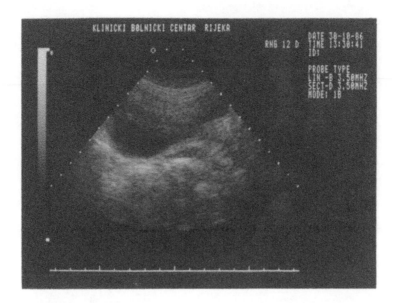

FIGURE 12.   Suprapubic longitudinal sector scan of chronic vesiculitis (note the thickened hyperechogenic vesicle wall).

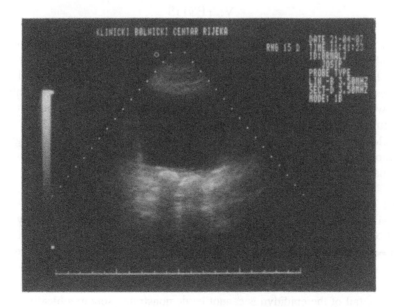

FIGURE 13.   Suprapubic transversal sector scan of both seminal vesicles with stone formations.

Congenital absence of the spermatic cord is very rare and is connected with cystic fibrosis. Iatrogenic injury of the vas deferens (herniorrhaphia, orchidopexia) sometimes can cause complete occlusion.

In normal subjects, the spermatic cord is not demonstrated by ultrasound. Acute inflammatory process of the testis spreads into the inguinal channel via the vas deferens and surrounding connective tissue. This process induces an enlargement and edema of the spermatic cord which is possible to recognize on sonolaminograms. Such pathological changes are present on sonograms as a band-like formation through the inguinal channel, surrounded by thin hypoechogenic boundaries due to inflammatory edema (Figure 14).

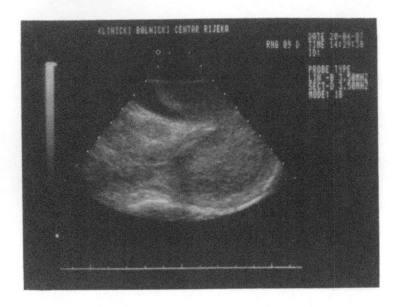

FIGURE 14.   Longitudinal sector scan on the level of the scrotal neck with the presentation of acute orchiepididymitis with vasitis.

V. TESTIS

Although the testis is an easily accessible organ for palpation, inflammatory changes, which are always associated with edema and pain, make detailed physical examinations impossible. However, radiologic diagnostic procedures (deferentography, epididymography, radioisotopes, etc.) may be useful for diagnosis in such cases, but they are, unfortunately, associated with complications. In recent years, ultrasound diagnosis of numerous diseases of the scrotum has been reported extensively.[12-17]

The development of high-resolution units with special transducers permits high quality of the sonographic image, so that sonography comes in first place among diagnostic methods of scrotal diseases.

A. Normal Testis

Normal size of the testis, as estimated by sonographic assessment of healthy volunteers, is 3.8 × 3 × 2.5 cm. The testis is denoted on sonograms as a homogeneous structure with a medium echogenicity of the testicular parenchyma. In the upper pole, it can be seen as an irregular area of hyperechogenicity which corresponds to the testicular net. The epididymis is more echogenic than the testicular parenchyma and, usually, the head of the epididymis is visible. The tail of the epididymis cannot be demonstrated sonographically in 20 to 40% of cases, and a small quantity of liquid surrounding the testis may be seen in 86% of cases. The thickness of the scrotal skin is 2 to 8 mm (Figure 15).

B. Acute Inflammatory Diseases

Acute inflammatory testicular and epididymal diseases may influence the number and motility of spermatozoa and the quantity of ejaculate, or cause strictures on the vasoepididymal connection. The existence of azoospermia and the inadequacy of ejaculate are accepted indications for performing the testicular biopsy. Some complications of acute orchiepididymitis, such as fibrosis, abscess formations, and diffuse suppuration, can extremely damage testicular function. Inflammatory lesions of the vasa and epididymis may be corrected by epididymovasostomy.

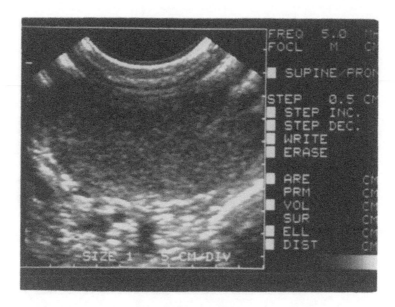

FIGURE 15.   Axial sector scan of a normal testis.

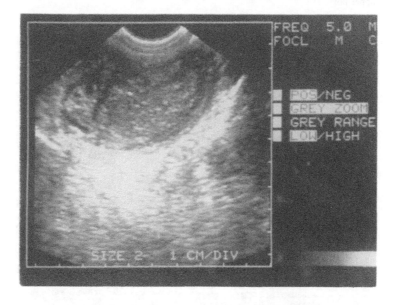

FIGURE 16.   Axial sector scan of acute orchiepididymitis.

1. Acute Orchiepididymitis

Acute orchitis very rarely shows up as an isolated inflammatory disease (mumps orchitis). It is mainly accompanied by epididymitis. With routine use of sonographs, an enlargement of the testicular parenchyma with irregular internal hypoechogenicity, which corresponds to the degree of the inflammatory edema, can be noticed. By regression of the inflammation, the quantity of internal echoes increases. Appearance of the focal anechogenic zone strongly suggests the development of an abscess formation, and such a sonographic feature indicates urgent surgical treatment (Figures 16 and 17).

2. Acute Epididymitis

Acute epididymitis is not unusual in urologic praxis. Chronic urinary tract infection,

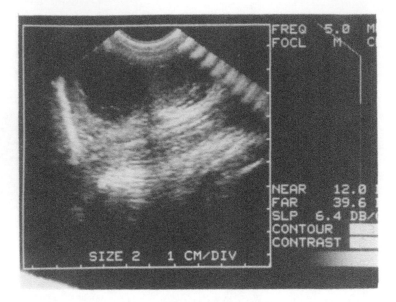

FIGURE 17.   Axial sector scan of a testis with a huge abscess formation in the upper pole.

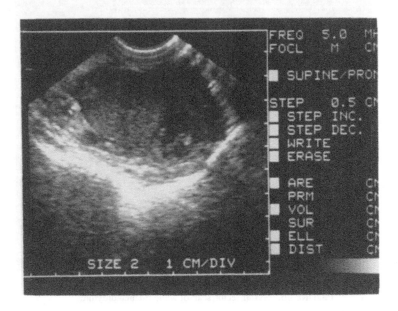

FIGURE 18.   Axial sector scan of a normal testis with acute epididymitis.

particularly prostatitis, and seminal vesiculitis, facilitates spreading of bacterial infection into the vasa deferentia and epididymis. Sonograms demonstrate normal echogenicity of the testicular parenchyma, while the epididymis is enlarged, sometimes greater than the testis, and has an irregular internal hypoechoic structure (Figure 18). The abscesses of the testis or epididymis have various sonographic findings. The ultrasound feature directly corresponds to the degree of pyogenic collection development (Figures 18 and 19).

C. Chronic Inflammatory Diseases

1. Chronic Epididymitis

Chronic epididymitis is shown on sonograms as an irregular hyperechoic band area ''be-

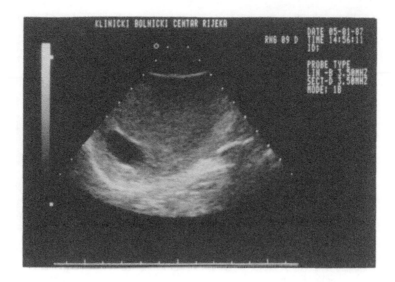

FIGURE 19. Axial sector scan of a normal testis with a small epididymal abscess.

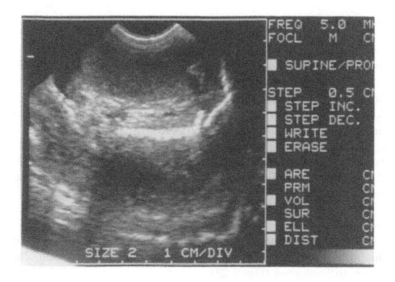

FIGURE 20. Axial sector scan of a normal testis with chronic epididymitis and small hydrocele.

hind'' the normal testis, and sonographic diagnosis must be confirmed in two basic scans. A diverse amount of fluid can be found in the scrotal sack (Figure 20).

2. Chronic Exacerbated Epididymitis

In the case of acute exacerbation of chronic epididymitis, the sonographic findings are completely changed. Within the hyperechoic epididymis, an irregular hypoechogenic area appears with progression of the disease, and corresponds to the inflammatory edema (Figure 21).

Both of these chronic diseases may be the underlying cause of inadequate spermatozoic maturation or mechanical obstruction development.

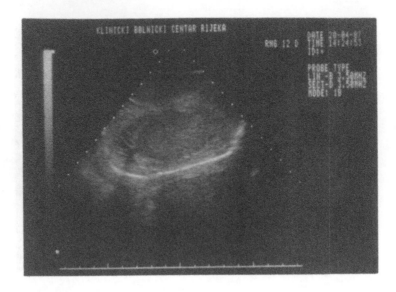

FIGURE 21.   Longitudinal sector scan of a normal testis with chronic exacerbated epididymitis.

D. Other Testicular Diseases

1. Varicocele

A dilatation of pampiniform plexus (varicocele) causes defective spermatogenesis, because of increased intrascrotal temperature. Varicocelectomy or ligature of the spermatic vein has been advocated in treatment of oligospermia.

Identification of the spermatic vein, in the spermatic cord at the scrotal neck, could be sonographically visible in each patient. On the longitudinal testicular scans, the dilatation of spermatic veins is seen as a tortuous hypoechoic area. Usually it consists of more than three veins, while at least one of them is more than 3 mm wide. The diagnosis is confirmed by an increase in vein size with the patient standing in the upright position or during Valsalva's maneuver.[3] The usefulness of Doppler studies in the diagnosis of subclinical varicoceles has also been reported (Figure 22).[18]

2. Pachyvaginitis

Chronic hyperthropic inflammation of the tunica albuginea of the testis can also affect the deferential duct, causing strictures or complete mechanical obstruction. The etiology of this condition is still unknown (Figure 23).

3. Pyocele

Secondary bacterial infection of the hydrocele or primary development of the pyocele can be very rare — the reason for extended infection along the spermatic cord (Figure 24). Characteristic sonographic features of the pyocele show irregularities of the inner scrotal layer and the presence of internal echoes within the anechogenic hydrocele. Such sonographic findings indicate an immediate operative treatment.

E. Testicular Trauma

Evaluation of the testical after traumatic injuries by ultrasound is relatively simple. Comparison to the usually normal, contralateral testis allows rapid identification of the abnormal architecture.[19]

Moreover, the sonographic finding helps in the final therapeutic approach (conservative or operative treatment). Usually, there are three types of testicular injuries.

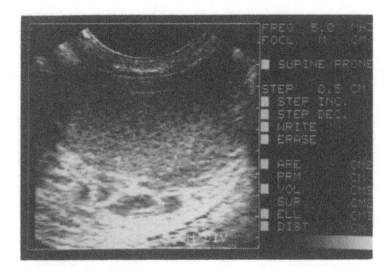

FIGURE 22. Longitudinal sector scan of a normal testis with presentation of a varicocele, placed posteriorly.

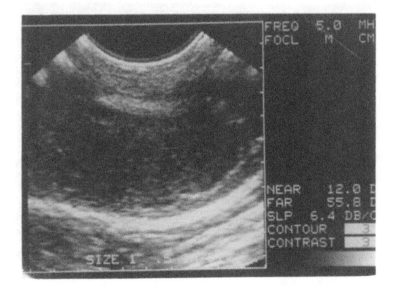

FIGURE 23. Axial sector scan with presentation of normal testicular tissue, surrounded with pachyvaginitis.

1. Testicular Rupture

Intratesticular rupture shows a swollen testis with regular boundaries. Hypoechogenic areas can be seen within the testicular tissue. In such cases, conservative treatment is recommended. The type of operative treatment depends on the place of rupture. The correct preoperative diagnosis of the ruptured testicle is possible to perform with ultrasound, and sonograms can help the surgeon in selection of operation type (simple sutures, partial resection, or semicastration) (Figure 25).

Early surgical intervention can save the testicular function. In most cases, traumatic

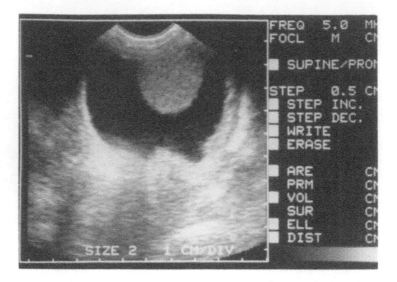

FIGURE 24. Transversal sector scan of a normal testis with a pyocele.

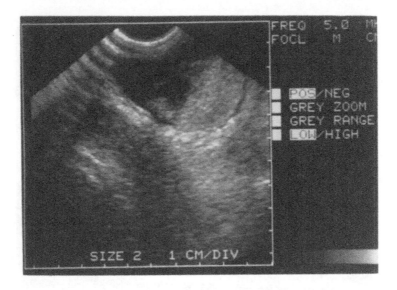

FIGURE 25. Longitudinal sector scan of an upper testicular pole rupture.

damage of the testiculoepididymal connection leads to complete obstruction with unilateral azoospermia.

2. Hematocele

Sonographic feature of the hematocele depends on maturation of the intrascrotal hematoma. Finally, the hydrocele is formed with fibrin bands within the scrotal sack. In the early period, after injury, the thickened scrotal skin and the anechogenic band surrounding the normal testis provide a typical picture of the simple hematocele (Figure 26).

Operative treatment is indicated in cases where the volume of the intrascrotal content is

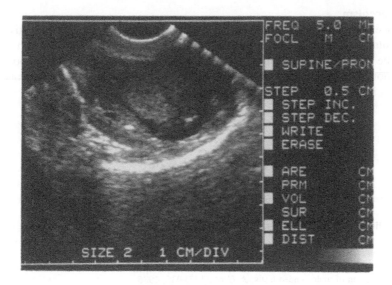

FIGURE 26.   Axial sector scan with hematocele and thickened edematous scrotal skin after blunt testicular trauma.

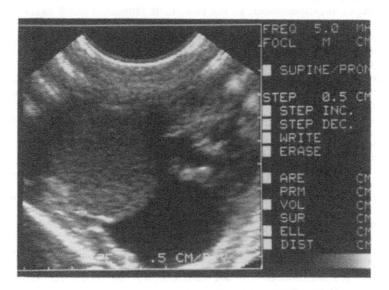

FIGURE 27.   Transversal sector scan of a normal testis with hydrocele rupture.

increased or clinical symptoms of secondary infection are present. By performing an operation based on repeated sonographic examinations, the complete testicular function is saved.

3. Rupture of Hydrocele

Over 60% of the normal population have a small amount of fluid within the scrotal neck. After blunt testicular trauma, the isolated rupture of the parietal tunica vaginalis can cause intrascrotal bleeding. Sonographically, the normal testis is surrounded by a fresh hematocele. The place of rupture is detectable by a sonography (Figure 27).

F. Kryptorchism

Maldescended testes occur in 0.7 to 0.8% of the child population. Preoperative diagnosis and testicular localization are necessary for planning the operative treatment. The retentioned testis in the inguinal channel is detected by ultrasound. The intra-abdominal position of the testis cannot be demonstrated during the sonographic examination and the "empty" inguinal channel on sonograms indicates the use of testicular venography.

REFERENCES

1. **Jimenez-Cruz, J. F., Mayayo, T., Lovaco, F., Garcia, J., Navio, S., and Romero-Acuirre, C.,** Transabdominal sonography of seminal vesicles, *J. Urol.,* 127, 260, 1982.
2. **Peeling, W. B. and Griffiths, G. J.,** Imaging of the prostate by ultrasound, *J. Urol.,* 132, 217, 1984.
3. **McClure, R. D. and Hricak, H.,** Scrotal ultrasound in the infertile man: detection of subclinical unilateral and bilateral varicoceles, *J. Urol.,* 135, 711, 1986.
4. **Weiss, R. M., Carter, A. R., and Rosenfield, A. T.,** High resolution real-time ultrasonography in the localisation of undescended testis, *J. Urol.,* 135, 936, 1986.
5. **Hennenberry, M., Carter, M. F., and Neiman, H. L.,** Estimation of prostate size by suprapubic ultrasonography, *J. Urol.,* 121, 615, 1979.
6. **Fuchkar, Z., Dimec, D., and Peterković, V.,** Transrectal sector sonography in prostatic disease, *Urol. Arch.,* 26, 135, 1986.
7. **Hastak, C. M., Gammelgaard, J., and Holn, H. H.,** Ultrasound guided transperineal biopsy in the diagnosis of prostatic carcinoma, *J. Urol.,* 128, 69, 1982.
8. **Fuchkar, Z.,** Transabdominal and transrectal sonography of seminal vesicles, *Medicina,* 22, 127, 1986.
9. **Tanahashi, Y., Watanabe, H., Igari, D., Harada, K., and Saitoh, M.,** Volume estimation of seminal vesicles by means of transrectal ultrasonomatography, *Br. J. Urol.,* 47, 695, 1975.
10. **Walls, W. and Linn, F.,** Ultrasonic diagnosis of seminal vesicle cyst, *Radiology,* 114, 693, 1975.
11. **Puigvert, A., Jimenez, J. F., Abos, P., and Cortes, F.,** Ureter ectopico en vesicula seminal, *Anal. Fund. Puigvert,* 6, 149, 1976.
12. **Miskin, B., Buckspan, M., and Bain, J.,** Ultrasonographic examination of scrotal masses, *J. Urol.,* 117, 185, 1977.
13. **Gottesman, J. E., Sample, W. F., Skinner, D. G., and Erlich, R. M.,** Diagnostic ultrasound in the evaluation of scrotal masses, *J. Urol.,* 118, 601, 1977.
14. **Blei, L., Scholnik, S., Bloom, D., Stutzman, R., and Chiodis, J.,** Ultrasonographic analysis of chronic intratesticular pathology, *J. Ultrasound Med.,* 2, 17, 1983.
15. **Carrol, B. A. and Gross, D. M.,** High-frequency scrotal sonography, *Am. J. Roentgenol.,* 140, 511, 1983.
16. **Leung, M. L., Gooding, G. A. W., and Williams, R. D.,** High-resolution sonography of scrotal contents in asymptomatic subjects, *Am. J. Roentgenol.,* 143, 161, 1984.
17. **Fuchkar, Z. and Dimec, D.,** Sonographic diagnosis of inflammatory diseases of the testis, *Urol. Arch.,* 26, 25, 1986.
18. **Greenberg, S. H., Lipshultz, L. I., and Wein, A. J.,** A preliminary report on "subclinical varicocele": diagnosis by Doppler ultrasonic stethoscope. Examination and initial results of surgical therapy, *J. Reprod. Med.,* 22, 77, 1979.
19. **Albert, N. E.,** Testicular ultrasound for trauma, *J. Urol.,* 124, 558, 1980.

INDEX

A

Printed and bound by CPI Group (UK) Ltd, Croydon, CR0 4YY

23/10/2024

01778245-0007